CONGENITAL DEFECTS
New Directions in Research

BIRTH DEFECTS INSTITUTE SYMPOSIA

Ernest B. Hook, Dwight T. Janerich, and Ian H. Porter, editors:
MONITORING, BIRTH DEFECTS AND ENVIRONMENT:
The Problem of Surveillance, 1971

Ian H. Porter and Richard G. Skalko, editors: HEREDITY AND
SOCIETY, 1972

Dwight T. Janerich, Richard G. Skalko, and Ian H. Porter, editors:
CONGENITAL DEFECTS: New Directions in Research, 1973

In preparation
Hilaire J. Meuwissen et al., editors:
COMBINED IMMUNOLOGICAL DISEASE: A Molecular Defect?, 1974

ACADEMIC PRESS RAPID MANUSCRIPT REPRODUCTION

CONGENITAL DEFECTS
New Directions in Research

Edited by

Dwight T. Janerich
Richard G. Skalko
Ian H. Porter

Assistant Editor

Sally Kelly

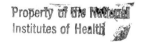

Birth Defects Institute
New York State Department of Health
Albany, New York

Proceedings of a Symposium on
Congenital Defects: New Directions in Research
Sponsored by the Birth Defects Institute of the
New York State Department of Health
Held in Albany, New York, October 30-31, 1972

Academic Press, Inc.
New York and London
A Subsidiary of Harcourt Brace Jovanovich, Publishers
1974

ACADEMIC PRESS, INC.
111 Fifth Avenue, New York, New York 10003

United Kingdom Edition published by
ACADEMIC PRESS, INC. (LONDON) LTD.
24/28 Oval Road, London NW1

LIBRARY OF CONGRESS CATALOG CARD NUMBER: 73-2080

PRINTED IN THE UNITED STATES OF AMERICA

CONTENTS

SECTION I

SECTION II

SECTION III

CONTENTS

CONTENTS

PARTICIPANTS

J. William Flynt, Jr., Center for Disease Control, Atlanta, Georgia

F. Clarke Fraser, McGill University, Montreal, Quebec, Canada

Peter Greenwald, Cancer Control Bureau, New York State Department of Health, Albany, New York

Alan R. Hinman, Epidemiology and Preventive Health Services, New York State Department of Health, Albany, New York

Ernest B. Hook, Birth Defects Institute, New York State Department of Health, Albany, New York

Dwight T. Janerich, Birth Defects Institute, New York State Department of Health, Albany, New York

Kenneth P. Johnson, Case Western Reserve University School of Medicine, Cleveland, Ohio

Sally M. Kelly, Birth Defects Institute, New York State Department of Health, Albany, New York

Frances O. Kelsey, Food and Drug Administration, Washington, D. C.

K. Sune Larsson, Karolinska Institute, Stockholm, Sweden

William M. Layton, Dartmouth Medical School, Hanover, New Hampshire

Abraham M. Lilienfeld, Johns Hopkins University, Baltimore, Maryland

Walter E. Nance, Indiana University, Indianapolis, Indiana

James V. Neel, University of Michigan, Ann Arbor, Michigan

Howard N. Newcombe, Atomic Energy of Canada Limited, Chalk River, Ontario, Canada

Ian H. Porter, Director, Birth Defects Institute, New York State Department of Health, Albany, New York

FOREWORD

This volume is a record of the third symposium held in Albany, New York on October 30 and 31, 1972, sponsored by the Birth Defects Institute of the New York State Department of Health.

This third symposium was attended by 325 registrants from 23 states and three foreign countries. This is the largest registration ever, more than double last year's. This gratifying attendance is in part a tribute to the Institute's staff who planned well and chose the participants and subjects wisely. But it is also a testimony to the mounting interest in birth defects among the scientific community.

There is so much that we do not know about this complex subject and we all agree it is a fascinating and promising field for scientific investigation. Since 1967, when the Institute was created by legislative action, it has been engaged in investigations into the causes and possible treatment of birth defects. It seeks to discover new environmental agents that may cause birth defects and to develop ways of making genetic counseling more effective. Three Institute staff members presented papers at this symposium describing some of the avenues that we are exploring. But I would like to call your attention to the fact that the heads of two other units of the New York State Health Department also participated in the program, which I think demonstrates that our concern for congenital defects is by no means limited to the work of the Birth Defects Institute.

Each year the proceedings of these symposia are published in order that the health professionals who are engaged in the field of birth defects can benefit from our efforts. This volume is intended to provide stimulation for the development of new areas in birth defects research, and I am sure that this collection of scientific material will accomplish that goal.

Hollis S. Ingraham, M. D.
Commissioner
New York State Department of Health
Albany, New York

ACKNOWLEDGMENTS

The Symposium upon which this volume is based could not have taken place without the expert administrative efforts of Edwin C. Jones and the support of the entire Birth Defects Institute staff. The skilled support which Ellen Heenehan, Sylvia Sickles, and Louise Skalko provided to the editors has been invaluable. To all these people we wish to express our sincere thanks and appreciation.

SECTION I

SECTION 1

A NOTE ON CONGENITAL DEFECTS IN TWO UNACCULTURATED INDIAN TRIBES

James V. Neel*

To a rough approximation, the precise etiology of approximately 80 percent of what we class as congenital malformations remains unclear. We cannot hope to develop a sound program of preventive measures — or define the limits within which preventive measures will have to operate — without a better understanding of etiology.

THE FREQUENCY OF MAJOR CONGENITAL DEFECTS IN DIVERSE POPULATIONS

One approach to etiology is the study of comparative teratology. How do the frequencies and types of major defects differ among populations living in widely different environments, where genetic background, disease pressures and diet differ widely?

In 1958, we published the first detailed comparison of the pattern of malformations in representatives of two very different ethnic groups with quite different life styles.[1] In a series of 64,569 births in Hiroshima, Kuré and Nagasaki during the years 1948 to 1954 (close to a total sample), 660 (1.02%) terminated in infants (live-or stillborn) with major congenital defects detected on physical examination. In Hiroshima, autopsies were performed on 62.8 percent of stillborn infants and infants dying during the neonatal period; on the basis of these findings, the frequency of congenital defect in the study population was estimated to be 1.34 percent. Excluded from that series are children whose parents received significant amounts of radiation at the time of the atomic bombings, and also children whose parents were consanguineous. I shall finesse the whole difficult question of what constitutes a major defect with the simple statement that we published our findings in detail; he who is motivated can inspect the list.

*The collection of these data was made possible by the financial support of the U.S. Atomic Energy Commission.

There was only one other series from Japan with which these results could be compared, the experience of the Red Cross Maternity Hospital in Tokyo, as summarized by Mitani.[2] There is an important source of potential bias in those data, in that in that period in Japan the greatest majority of births either occurred at home, attended by midwives, or in the private facilities of mid-wives. One could suspect that the Red Cross Hospital attracted complicated labors, in which the percentage of malformed fetuses could be unusually high. Nevertheless, the frequency of 0.92 percent published by Mitani agrees very well with our own (Mitani's series excluded congenital heart disease).

At that time, I made a rather careful survey of the literature on the subject based on Caucasian births. It was — and remains — a most uneven literature. However, in eight series of Caucasian births where the procedures and criteria seemed similar to those employed in Japan, the nonweighted average frequency of major congenital defect was 1.20 percent. The fraction of children coming to autopsy is difficult to determine. This is very similar to the Japanese figure and I concluded that when attention is restricted to carefully collected series, there was an impressive constancy in the total frequency of major congenital defects in diverse groups. This similarity between Mongolians (predominantly Chinese and Japanese ancestry) and Caucasians in frequency of major defects persists in Hawaii.[3] While I don't doubt that someday a Caucasian series will be found which differs "significantly" from the Japanese, to me the impressive finding is the similarity. In passing, we should note that this impression of relative constancy is based only upon those fetuses surviving five months; there is an urgent need for data on early fetal loss.

However, although the total impact of congenital defect on Japanese and Caucasian populations was very similar, the incidence of specific defects varied significantly (Table 1). The two most striking examples were harelip with or without cleft palate and defects of the central nervous system, the former being 54 percent more frequent in Japanese but the latter 154 percent more frequent in the Caucasian series.

SOME GENETIC CONSIDERATIONS

This relative constance of total impact in the face of widely varying diet and disease patterns, although the frequency of specific defects varied widely, struck me as a finding demanding explanation. How was it that two very different populations exhibited about the same frequency of congenital defect when they differed so widely in respect to a variety of other aspects of their patterns of disease? It is clear that the etiology of congenital defect is complex and heterogeneous, but is it a sufficient working hypothesis to postulate that somehow, in very different ethnic groups, chance mixes of genetic and environ-

TABLE 1

Frequency of Occurrence of Six Readily Diagnosed Malformations in Japanese and Caucasian Births, After Neel (1958)

Population	Location	Investigator	No. of Births	Defect												Total Dx.	Dx. per 1,000 children
				anencephaly		spina bifida		anoph-microph-thalmos		atresia ani		harelip-cleft palate		polydactyly			
				no.	incidence	no.	incidence	no.	incidence	no.	incidence	no.	incidence	no.	incidence		
Japanese	This series	This series	63,796	40	0.00063	13	0.00020	16	0.00025	15	0.00024	171	0.00268	59	0.00092	314	4.92
	Tokyo	Mitani, 1943	49,645	33	0.00066	11	0.00022	10	0.00020	15	0.30030	94	0.00189	57	0.00115	220	4.43
		Total	113,441	73	0.00064	24	0.00021	26	0.00023	30	0.30026	265	0.00234	116	0.00102	534	
Caucasian	England	Malpas, 1937	13,964	44	0.00315	39	0.00279	0	– – –	4	0.00029	17	0.00122	16*	0.00115	120	8.59
	Switzerland	Ehrat, 1948	50,147	27	0.00054	54	0.00108	6†	0.00012	20	0.00040	74	0.00148	20	0.00040	201	4.01
	U.S.A.	Lucy, 1949	11,881	13	0.00109	15	0.00126	0	– – –	1	0.00008	15	0.00126	9	0.00076	53	4.46
	Sweden	Böök, 1951	44,109	24	0.00054	47	0.00107	4	0.00009	19	0.00043	77	0.00175	30	0.00068	201	4.56
		Total	120,101	108	0.00090	155	0.00129	10	0.00008	44	0.00037	183	0.00152	75	0.00062	575	

*Entered as "malformed hands and arms"; undoubtedly includes more than polydactyly.

†The author lists 12 cases of "Missbildungen des äusseren Ohres, der Nase, der Augen". On the basis of our experience in Japan, it has been estimated that not more than half of these fall into the anophthalmos-microphthalmos category. This rough approximation, made necessary by the grouping of the data, probably fixes the upper limit of the frequency of the defect.

mental effects just happen to mesh in such a way as to produce similar total frequencies of major defect? In a search for a unifying principle, as a tentative hypothesis for some fraction of congenital defect, I suggested that "many congenital malformations of various types find a partial explanation in the existence in man of genetic systems of the type discussed in such penetrating and provocative detail by Lerner..., 'the malformations (phenodeviants) being caused by the intrinsic properties of multigenic Mendelian inheritance, due to which a certain percentage of individuals of every generation falls below the threshold of the obligate proportion of loci needed in a heterozygous state to ensure normal development.' The similarity in malformation frequencies in such diverse populations as Japanese and European thus finds an explanation in the fact that there is a malformation frequency representing the optimum balance between, on the one hand, fetal loss and physical handicap from congenital defect and, on the other hand, population gain from those very same genes which in certain combinations may sometimes result in physical defect".[1]

This suggestion was not received with universal approbation and there has followed a rather lively exchange, recently summarized in Schull and Neel.[4] It is admittedly a difficult hypothesis to test cleanly. Let me say only that I regard the recent emergence of the concept that some human congenital defects should be regarded as examples of quasi-continuous variation with a threshold effect[5,6,7] as an endorsement of the suggestion of an effect of homozygosity *per se,* albeit limited to one end of the distribution curve for homozygosity. This latter concept clearly demands that the same phenotype result from a variety of genotypes which have in common the same degree of homozygosis for the multifactorial system concerned.

Two lines of evidence make it clear that the expression of those postulated genetic systems in any one individual is delicately balanced. Firstly, concordance rates for most congenital defects are rather low in identical twins, and this was true in our own series. Secondly, there is evidence for seasonal, secular and maternal age and parity effects for a number of malformations. Most studied in this respect are congenital defects of the central nervous system. McKeown and Record,[8] using data from Birmingham, England and all Scotland for 1939-1947, first developed a provocative case for seasonal variation in the frequency of anencephaly (but not hydrocephalus or spina bifida), from 1.9/1000 births in May to 3.1/1000 births in December. Since a contrast between the low and high months may be unduly influenced by sampling error, it seems more conservative to contrast the low half of the year (2.2/1000 with the high half, 2.8/1000). However, these effects, although significant, were minor in contrast to ethnic differences in

6

the frequency of this defect.   However, the possibility of more major environmental factors now emerges from the epidemiological studies of Yen and McMahon,[9] Naggan[10] and Rogers and Morris.[11]

On the other hand, delicate balance or not, I find it very thought-provoking how similar the malformation picture of the American Indian is to the Japanese.   Adams and Niswander[12] report a total major malformation frequency of 1.86 percent in 18,811 hospital-born U.S. Indian infants.   Their list seems to include some diagnoses that can only be confirmed by autopsy, so that their frequency is perhaps best compared with our figure of 1.34 percent.   The Indians, like the Japanese, show relatively low frequencies of anencephaly and spina bifida.   However, while the frequency of isolated cleft palate is strikingly similar in Japanese and Indians, harelip with or without cleft palate has in Indians a frequency intermediate between Japanese and Caucasians.[13,14,1] Evidently the different environment of the new world has altered the mongoloid pattern of congenital defect relatively little; it is difficult not to see genetic implications in this observation.

There has been a massive accumulation of data on the frequency of congenital defects since that 1958 paper, although there is still a real paucity of data on native African populations.   This literature has been reviewed by a number of authors;[15,16,17] there is no need to re-review it now.   It still appears that congenital defects have a very similar impact on all properly studied populations.

A variety of congenital defects, of vision and hearing, or mental deficiency, are readily missed at birth.   There has been a need for series of children followed well into childhood.   There are now two series on physical defects in cohorts of Caucasian children followed for some time after birth[18,19] and we have published two follow-ups on a subset of our earlier material.[20] McIntosh et al.[18] recorded that 6.3 percent of a cohort of 3,101 white children followed from birth to an average age of 1 year had some type of congenital defect, whereas for 2,429 non-white children the corresponding figure was 7.8 percent.   The examination of these children included extensive radiological studies not pursued in our series.   Elsewhere, I have reviewed their data and concluded that by the standards we employed, and if the common defect of polydactyly in the Negro was excluded from consideration, their figure would approximate 5 percent.[1]

McKeown and Record[19] reported the results of a five-year study of a cohort identified in Birmingham, England.   For a group of 8 readily identifiable congenital malformations, the frequency in the cohort of 56,760 was 1.7 percent on the basis of an examination at birth, and 2.3 percent on the basis of the five-year follow-up.

In our data from Japan, among 16,144 children examined at birth and again (if alive) at 9 months, the frequency of major congenital defect was recorded at 3.12 percent.[1] McKeown and Record[19] compared the Birmingham and Japanese data with respect to those eight defects mentioned earlier, finding our frequency for these specific defects to be 2.4%. They comment that although the total frequencies are very similar, the specific types vary considerably in frequency. Among 3,570 children examined at birth and again (if alive) at an average age of 8½ years, the frequency of "significant" defect, probably congenital in nature, was 5.5 percent.[20] We have published a detailed listing of these defects, so that another investigator can "adjust" our list as he sees fit.

There are the usual problems of consistency between series, which can only be solved when investigators are prepared to publish their results in detail (and can persuade editors that this is the way it must be done). For the present, my impression is that the frequency of significant defect, congenital in origin, in a cohort of Japanese and Caucasian children followed well into childhood is about the same.

At this point, I must take exception to one aspect of the otherwise excellent review of Lilienfeld.[16] In Table 1 he gives the range of congenital defect in diverse populations as 1.02 to 12.33 percent. The 1.02 is drawn from my paper, the 12.33 from Farrer and Mackie.[21] Curious to learn more about this epidemic, I went to the original source, which opens with this sentence: "The present survey was initiated by the staff of the Southerland District Hospital because an unusually high number of abnormal babies was born in the hospital during the months of September and October, 1961." In fact, over a period of one year there were 24 congenitally defective children among a total of 1,865 births; 13 of these were born in September and October. This classical demonstration of biased figures scarcely needed a 10-fold inflation by a misplaced decimal point!

Special reference must be made to the rather ambitious effort of Stevenson et al.[22] to collect world-wide data, from maternity services in 24 population centers. Exclusive of malformations of the heart, talipes and congenital dysplasia of the hip, the reported frequency of major defect at birth varied among single births from 2.6/1000 in Calcutta to 16.3/1000 in Belfast. If valid, these differences would seem to refute the hypothesis of relative constancy of major defect in widely different ethnic groups. The authors discuss at length the problem of obtaining uniform diagnostic standards in all centers. Some insight into this problem may be gained from the data from Bombay, where 340 (.86 percent) among 39,498 births in five hospitals were reported with major defects. It so happened that simultaneously an independent study was in progress at the hospital which provided the major source of these data, in which all newborns were checked by one person. This

8

study yielded a figure of 420 defects (1.58 percent) among 26,631 single births.[23,24] The authors distinguish between births occurring to women registered in the clinic and births to women seen at the hospital for the first time at the termination of the pregnancy. The frequency with which defective children were born in the latter situation (2.9 percent) is twice the frequency in the former (1.4 percent), illustrating once again a well-known source of bias at work. For three defects where no diagnostic problems should arise, the frequencies per 1000 were as follows:

	Stevenson et al. 1966[22]	Master-Notani et al. 1968[23]
Atresia ani without neural tube defect	0.38	0.75
Anencephaly with or without other defects	1.52	1.69
Polydactyly alone	0.38	1.65

The discrepancy illustrates once more the profound difficulties which still persist in the reporting of congenital defects.

OBSERVATIONS ON UNACCULTURATED AMERICAN INDIANS

Against this background, I come finally to the subject of my presentation, congenital malformations among primitive peoples. We have for the past 10 years been involved in studies of two of the most primitive tribes of Indians still to be found in South America, the Xavante and the Yanomama. They *are* primitive, pursuing still a life style about as different from our own as can be imagined. I believe you will agree they would constitute a severe test of the thesis of the relative constancy of the total impact of congenital defect.

These Indians live in small villages, few of which are in contact with qualified observers. Births are usually in the bush; malformed infants are often killed. What we see when we conduct physical examinations on entire villages are the survivors of a severe selective process. Thus, our findings represent absolutely minimal figures. Having been critical of the data of others, I now wish clearly to label our own observations as a non-series, never to be used for normative purposes.

We have by now examined in a systematic fashion 287 Xavante and 513

Yanomama of all ages, from 10 different villages[25,26,27] (Oliver and Neel, unpublished). These are, on the average, young populations, the estimated average age being in the mid-twenties. The congenitally malformed persons we detect must first have escaped infanticide and they must then have survived in the harsh environment until we came upon the scene. Table 2 summarizes the major malformations encountered which should have been detectable at birth. The bulk of that total figure of 14 is contributed by one single entry, congenital heart disease, type undetermined. The definitive diagnosis of congenital heart disease now depends on elaborate X-ray studies, including cardiac catheterization, none available to us. Our diagnosis rests solely on physical examinations, for which the responsibility was shared by three pediatricians and myself. The findings, to be presented in detail elsewhere, were in most instances those that in a U.S. setting we would associate with congenital heart disease or, less probably, rheumatic heart disease but, of course, we cannot exclude some exotic causation. No cases of rheumatic fever have been observed in either of these groups. From appropriate antibody studies on the Xavante, it has been concluded that: "On the basis of a U.S. experience, the distribution of streptococcal antibody titers in this population suggests sporadic exposure to mild streptococcal infection of some type."[28] Similar antibody titers were encountered in the Yanomama and, in addition, 14 of 55 throat cultures yielded β-hemolytic streptococcus (Moody and Neel, unpublished). Thus, the possibility of rheumatic fever is real. It is noteworthy that in 9 of the 11 presumptive diagnoses, the murmurs were limited to systole, usually best heard in the left second or third interspaces, and were felt most suggestive of auricular or ventricular septal defect (with or without other anomalies).

If we attribute all of the cardiac findings to congenital heart disease, then we observe 14 congenitally defective persons among 800. Even if we attribute half of the cardiac findings to acquired disease, the figure is 9 out of 800. It seems best not to dignify this observation by calculating a quotable rate or incidence figure since, on the one hand, we may have hit an unusual "pocket" of congenital heart disease but, on the other hand, we are missing those defects incompatible with survival or resulting in infanticide. The possibility cannot be discarded that some unusual exogenous agent with rather specific effects on the developing heart is involved, comparable to the role of *Veratrum californicum* in a cyclopian-type deformity in lambs[29] or, if Renwick (this Symposium) is correct, the role of some potato-blight-associated factor in human anencephaly. We note in passing that in the data of Adams and Niswander[12] on the North American Indian, congenital heart disease, type undetermined, had a high frequency (0.40 percent, as contrasted to 0.14 percent in our Japanese series), and the Xavante and Yanomama may thus exhibit

TABLE 2

The Congenital Defects Recognizable at Birth Detected in an Unselected
Consecutive Series of 287 Xavante and 513 Yanomama Indians

Tribes	Types of Malformations	No. Cases
Xavante	Congenital heart disease	3
	Polydactyly	1
	Talipes equinovarus	1
Yanomama	Congenital heart disease	8 + 3 ?
	Spastic diplegia	1
		14 + 3 ?

a high degree of an 'Indian trait'. Incidentally, since congenital heart disease is not detected by inspection, such infants would not be killed — it must be regarded in a different light from the other defects.

There is one other small source of information, the observations of missionaries in intimate contact with the Yanomama. Between 1959 (when contacts were initiated) and 1967 (when we first visited the villages), missionaries in contact with two of the villages recorded the outcome of all pregnancies in the village whose termination was known to them. Among 93 terminations, four were probably characterized by congenital malformation: one stillborn described by the Indians as having one very short upper limb and other deformities; one killed because of deformity, not otherwise described; and two with encephalocoele. These latter were flown out to the territorial capital for surgery; one died shortly thereafter but the other survived and was seen by me.

We have, of course, also seen examples of congenital defect in villages not subjected to systematic examination. Noteworthy was the achondroplastic dwarf which we had observed. Although he obviously escaped infanticide at birth, presumably because the syndrome was not recognized, the Indians alleged that he had fathered a child, also achondroplastic, who was so recognized and killed at birth.

These observations, which suggest that the frequency of congenital defect among a primitive people is at least as great as among ourselves, and perhaps even greater, are so unsatisfactory that we have hesitated to put them on record. However, with the current interest in the epidemiology of congenital defect, perhaps we can stimulate others to come forward with, or to generate, similar data. The most nearly similar data known to me are those of Mann *et al.*,[30] who encountered significant heart murmurs in five of 292 Pygmies. I realize that in hinting at the possibility of a high frequency of at least some congenital defects among primitive populations, I am in danger of vitiating my earlier argument for the relative constancy of the total amount of congenital defect in all populations. This leads to one last comment; namely, that the rate of inbreeding is quite high among the Yanomama; from a computer simulation program based on the observed structure of four Yanomama villages, we estimate that the spouses in an average marriage are the genetic equivalent of first cousins once removed (MacCluer and Neel, unpublished). There is evidence that in some populations the frequency of congenital defect is increased in consanguineous marriages.[31,22] This factor must be considered in efforts at comparing the Yanomama with other populations.

CONCLUSION

In summary, it is sobering how many gaps there still are in our descriptive knowledge of human congenital defect, and how many conflicts must be resolved between what observations there are. The accumulation of good data on good teratology is a slow and not too exciting business, and it is tempting to leave it to the vital statistician and his birth certificates or look to hospital records for the answers. Unfortunately, this approach has not proved satisfactory in the past in studies of comparative teratology, nor will it provide badly needed data on congenital defects in foetuses lost early in pregnancy. There is, in particular, an urgent need for well-organized studies on primitive people to whom medical services are just being extended, since they represent extremes of environmental and nutritional adaptation which will not long be available for study, and since they provide a much needed baseline against which to evaluate the frequently discussed possible impact of "civilization" on this important cause of mortality and morbidity.

REFERENCES

1. J.V. Neel, *Amer. J. Hum. Genet. 10,* 398, 1958.

2. S. Mitani, *Gyn.& Obstet. 11,* 345, 1943.

3. N.E. Morton, *Am. J. Hum. Genet. 19,* 23, 1967.

4. W.J. Schull and J.V. Neel, *Am. J. Hum. Genet. 24,* 425, 1972.

5. C.O. Carter, *in* Progress in Medical Genetics, 4, A.G. Steinberg, A.G. Bearn, (Eds.), Grune & Stratton, New York, p. 59, 1965.

6. C.S. Chung, R.W. Nemechek, I.J. Larson and G.H.S. Ching, *Hum. Hered. 19,* 321, 1969.

7. C.M. Woolf, *J. Med. Genet. 8,* 65, 1971.

8. T. McKeown and R.G. Record, *Lancet I,* 192, 1951.

9. S. Yen and B. MacMahon, *Lancet II,* 623, 1968.

10. L. Naggan, *Amer. J. Epidemiol. 89,* 154, 1969.

11. S.C. Rogers and M. Morris, *Ann. Hum. Genet. 34,* 295, 1971.

12. M.S. Adams and J.D. Niswander, *Eugen.Quart. 15,* 227, 1968.

13. V.E. Tretsven, *J. Speech Hearing Dis. 28,* 52, 1963.

14. J.R. Miller, *in* Papers and Discussions presented at II Intern. Conf. on Congen. Malform., New York, M. Fishbein (Ed.), International Medical

Congress, Ltd., New York, p. 334, 1964.

15. M. Lamy and J. Frezel, *in* Papers and Discussions presented at I Intern. Conf. on Congen. Malform., London, M. Fishbein (Ed.), J.B. Lippincott Co., Philadelphia, p. 34, 1960.

16. A.M. Lilienfeld, *in* Congenital Malformations, F.C. Fraser and V.A. McKusick (Eds.), Excerpta Medica, Amsterdam, p. 251, 1970.

17. J. Warkany, *in* Congenital Malformations, Year Book Medical Publishers, Inc., Chicago, pp. *xi* and 1309, 1971.

18. R. McIntosh, K.K. Merritt, M.R. Richards, M.H. Samuels and M.T. Bellows, *Pediatrics 14*, 505, 1954.

19. T. McKeown and R.G. Record, *in* Ciba Foundation Symposium on Congenital Malformations, G.E.W. Wolstenholme and C.M. O'Connor (Eds.), Brown and Co., Boston, p. 2, 1960.

20. W.J. Schull and J.V. Neel, *in* The Effects of Inbreeding on Japanese Children, Harper and Row, New York, pp. *xii* and 419, 1965.

21. J.F. Farrer and I.J. Mackie, *Med. J. Aust. 2*, 702, 1964.

22. A.C. Stevenson, H.A. Johnston, M.I.P. Stewart and D.R. Golding, *in* Bull. World Health Organ., Suppl. 34, 127, 1966.

23. P. Master-Notani, P.J. Kolah and L.D. Sanghvi, *Acta. Genet. 18*, 97, 1968.

24. P.J. Kolah, P.A. Master and L.D. Sanghvi, *Amer. J. Obstet. Gynec. 97*, 400, 1967.

25. J.V. Neel, F.M. Salzano, P.C. Junqueira, F. Keiter and D. Maybury-Lewis, *Amer. J. Hum. Genet. 16*, 52, 1964.

26. E.D. Weinstein, J.V. Neel and F.M. Salzano, *Amer. J. Hum. Genet. 19*, 532, 1967.

27. H.P. Baker and J.V. Neel, *in* Abstracts of Contributed Papers,III Intern. Congr. Hum. Genet., Chicago, p. 4, 1966.

28. J.V. Neel, A.H.P. Andrade, G.E. Brown, W.E. Eveland, J. Goobar, W.A. Sodeman, G.H. Stollerman, E.D. Weinstein and A.H. Wheeler, *Amer. J. Trop. Med. Hyg. 17*, 486, 1968.

29. J.M. Robson, F.M. Sullivan and R.L. Smith, *in* Embryopathic Activity of Drugs, Little, Brown and Co., Boston, 1965.

30. G.V. Mann, O.A. Roels, D.L. Price and J.M. Merrill, *J. Chron. Dis. 15,* 341, 1962.

31. W.J. Schull, *Amer. J. Hum. Genet. 10*, 294,1958.

SOME ASPECTS OF MATERNAL EFFECTS ON CONGENITAL MALFORMATIONS

F. Clarke Fraser

In 1960, Anne McLaren[1] concluded a talk on maternal effects in mammals by saying: "Thus, the mammals have open to them an alternative pathway of inheritance, a somatic, maternal, non-chromosomal pathway.... To what extent mammals have availed themselves of this opportunity must await further research." I would like to suggest that such maternal effects are often found when looked for, and describe a number of examples drawn mainly from studies on gene-environment interactions, carried out in our laboratory over the past 20 years.

When we found that cortisone, injected into pregnant mothers, produced cleft palates in the offspring with different frequencies in the A/J (A-susceptible) and C57BL/6 (C-resistant) strains[2] (Table 1, lines 1 and 2), it seemed logical to begin a genetic analysis by crossing the two strains and testing the F1 hybrids. Somewhat to our surprise, we found a reciprocal cross difference,[3] the frequency in the F1 hybrids being higher when the susceptible strain was the mother (Table 1, lines 3 and 4). Appropriate backcrosses showed that this maternal effect was not cytoplasmically transmitted to the next generation.[4] Females from a cross between an A mother and a C father and mated to A males (AC x A) gave no higher frequencies of offspring with cleft palate than females from a cross of a C mother by an A father mated to A males (CA x A) (Table 1, lines 5 and 6). These back-cross offspring had similar genotypes but differed in the origin of any factors transmitted through the cytoplasm. We have no idea of the nature of the uterine differences involved, but they are correlated with differences in the gestational stage and rate at which the embryonic palates close,[5] so the maternal effect, as well as the embryonic genotype, seems to alter the cleft palate frequency by altering the timing of a normal developmental process. Whether this accounts for the entire reciprocal cross difference we do not know. Perhaps there is also some relation to the mother's failure to "justify" her hormones, in a manner suggested in Bessman's[6] recent intriguing hypothesis advanced with respect to inborn errors of amino acid metabolism.

17

TABLE 1

Some Examples of Maternal Effects on Genotypic Expression

(See text for explanation)

	Cross	Defect	Treatment	N	% Affected
1.	A x A	Cleft palate	Cortisone	36	100
2.	C x C	Cleft palate	Cortisone	86	17
3.	A x C	Cleft palate	Cortisone	46	43
4.	C x A	Cleft palate	Cortisone	82	4
5.	AC x A	Cleft palate	Cortisone	116	22
6.	CA x A	Cleft palate	Cortisone	71	25
7.	A x CA	Cleft lip	None	267	4
8.	CA x A	Cleft lip	None	640	0.2
9.	F x (CFxF)	Cleft lip	None	563	14
10.	(CFxF) x F	Cleft lip	None	404	5
11.	(FxCF) x F	Cleft lip	None	431	5
12.	A x A	Resorption	None	650	20
13.	C x C	Resorption	None	390	13
14.	C x A	Resorption	None	322	14
15.	CA x A	Resorption	None	640	5
16.	A x CA	Resorption	None	267	18
17.	C x C	Cleft palate	6AN 19mg/kg, L.C.	108	11
18.	C x C	Cleft palate	6AN 19mg/kg, B.C.	117	67
19.	A x A	Cleft palate	6AN 14mg/kg, L.C.	82	65
20.	A x A	Cleft palate	6AN 14mg/kg, B.C.	102	56
21.	CA x A	Cleft palate	6AN 19mg/kg, L.C.	295	26
22.	AC x A	Cleft palate	6AN 19mg/kg, B.C.	200	44
23.	CAA x A	Cleft palate	6AN 14mg/kg, L.C.	134	51
24.	ACA x A	Cleft palate	6AN 14mg/kg, L.C.	105	43

There was also an intriguing interaction with maternal weight. A females were more susceptible to a fixed dose of cortisone on one diet than another whereas C females reacted in the opposite direction, but only if the females weighed over 22 grams at conception.[7]

Of course, maternal effects are not limited to congenital defects induced by a teratogen; they may also influence spontaneous malformations. In an analysis of the genetic basis of spontaneous cleft lip in the A/J strain,[8] a series of back-crosses were performed in which embryos were gestated by A/J females and hybrid females at varying degrees of hybridity, using A/J fathers. In up to 6 back-cross generations, the cleft lip frequency was higher in mice of comparable genotype, gestated by A/J than by hybrid mothers. A variety of experiments failed to reveal the nature of the difference between the two uterine environments.

A series of crosses set up by Bornstein et al.[9] showed that the maternal effect on cleft frequency was not transmitted by the cytoplasm. In this experiment an inbred strain, CL/Fr, with a relatively high frequency of cleft lip (about 25%), was used instead of A/J. (This strain will be referred to as F in the table to avoid confusion with the C strain.) The maternal effect was again demonstrated (e.g., line 9 vs. line 10). Where the embryos are of comparable genotype the cleft lip frequency is higher when the mother is from the susceptible strain. The cross in line 10 differs from that in line 11 only in the origin of any presumed cytoplasmic transmissible factors, and there is no difference in cleft lip frequency.

Puzzlingly, attempts to confirm these maternal differences (which have been repeatedly demonstrated in crosses) by ova transfer, and by ovarian transplant have given negative results — the cleft lip frequency remains obstinately close to that predicted by its genotype and uninfluenced by a different uterine environment. A similar situation has been found by Dr. Larsson's group[10] with cortisone-induced cleft palate. Thus, the maternal effect seems to be cytoplasmic, in the sense that it appears to reside in the egg cytoplasm rather than the intra-uterine environment, but not cytoplasmic in the sense that it is transmitted to the next generation. However, there is some conflicting evidence[11] and we have not ruled out an interaction with fetal death (resorption).

In Davidson's experiment a maternal effect on spontaneous resorption was also observed. Hybrid embryos in an inbred mother (Table 1, line 14) were resorbed as frequently as inbred embryos in the same mothers (line 13). In the back-cross, resorption frequency was low in the offspring of the hybrid mother (line 15) but not for offspring of comparable genotype of an inbred mother (line 16).

When we turned to another teratogen, 6-aminonicotinamide, the same kind of matroclinous reciprocal difference as with cortisone was found, the A strain again being susceptible, and the C strain resistant.[12] However, the C strain was much more resistant when the mother was raised on Purina Lab Chow (high in niacin) than on Breeder Chow (lines 17 and 18), whereas the A/J strain did not show this difference in response to different diets (lines 19 and 20). To our surprise, this factor causing resistance produced by the Breeder Chow diet persisted into the first back-cross (lines 21 and 22), though it was not manifest when the mice were raised on Lab Chow.[13] It seems likely that the difference resides in the mitochondria, where the inactive NAD analog formed from 6AN interferes with oxidative phosphorylation, and preliminary attempts to relate the physical properties of the mitochondria with these strain differences appeared promising (Verrusio, unpublished).

The factor was not transmitted through the sperm, and did not persist into the second back-cross.[14] Table 1 (lines 23 and 24) shows that the embryos in which the postulated particles were transmitted, via the cytoplasm, from the C57 line (CAA x A) did not have a lower frequency of cleft palate than the comparable embryos lacking the particles (ACA x A). This may mean either that the postulated cytoplasmic factor accounting for the differences in the first back-cross does not persist indefinitely as in the case of the Dauermodification described by Jollos fifty years ago[15] – although the latter factors persisted for more than two generations. Alternatively, it could mean that the difference in response is not the result of a cytoplasmic factor transmitted to the treated embryo, but some effect on the treated mother of the uterine environment to which she was raised. Such a situation has been reported by Zamenhoff[16] who showed that a reduction in cerebral DNA caused by maternal protein deficiency persisted in the F2 from the F1 animals which were not themselves protein deficient.

Our results could be explained by postulating that the embryo's mitochondrial DNA was transcribed from the maternal genome and then amplified in a manner similar to that of the ribosomal RNA.[14] This would result in those characteristics of the mitochondria that depend on their DNA being determined by the maternal genotype. If it is further assumed that the diet-dependent difference in response to 6AN is determined by the mother's rather than the embryo's mitochondria one would expect the reciprocal cross difference in the F1 to persist in the first back-cross and disappear in the second back-cross. This is, of course, only speculation, but is as good an explanation as any other so far advanced.

Finally, one may ask whether maternal effects exist in man. Of course, there are the well known effects of maternal age and parity on quantitative characters such as birth weight, and the frequency of several kinds of congenital defects, and a cytoplasmic factor has been invoked as a predisposing cause of anencephaly and sireniform malformations.[17]

Alport's disease shows divergences from the expectation for Mendelian autosomal dominant inheritance that have evoked a variety of possible explanations, but which we find best accounted for by a maternal effect on the penetrance of the gene in males. That is, when a male inherits the gene from his father, and develops in the uterus of a normal mother, he has less chance of developing the disease than if he inherits the mutant gene from his mother and develops in an "affected" environment.[18] A similar situation has recently been suggested for early-onset dystrophia myotonica.[19]

In conclusion, it appears that maternal influences on genotypic expression are not uncommon, when looked for — we found those I have reported even without looking for them. There is evidence that they occur in man as well as mouse. They may be important, as guides to means of prevention of diseases and defects. The discovery of their biochemical nature provides an exciting goal for the future.

REFERENCES

1.   A. McLaren, *in* Proc. 1st Intern. Conf. on Congenital Malformations, Lippincott, Philadelphia, pp. 211–222, 1962.

2.   F.C. Fraser and T.D. Fainstat, *Pediatrics 7*, 527, 1951.

3.   F.C. Fraser, H. Kalter, B.E. Walker and T.D. Fainstat, *J. Cell. Comp. Physiol. 43*, Supp. 1, 237, 1954.

4.   H. Kalter, *Genetics 39 (2)*, 185, 1954.

5.   D.G. Trasler, *in* Teratology (Wilson/Warkany, Eds.), U. Chicago Press, pp. 38–55, 1965.

6.   S.P. Bessman, *J. Pediatr. 81*, 834, 1972.

7.   D. Warburton, D.G. Trasler, A. Naylor, J.R. Miller and F.C. Fraser, *Lancet II*, 1116, 1962.

8.   J.G. Davidson, F.C. Fraser and G. Schlager, *Teratology 2 (4)*, 371, 1969.

9.   S. Bornstein, D.G. Trasler and F.C. Fraser, *Teratology 3 (4)*, 295, 1970.

10.   L. Marsk, M. Theorell and K.S. Larsson, *Nature 234*, 358, 1971.

11.   K. Takano, A.C. Peterson, F.G. Biddle and J.R. Miller, *Teratology 5*, 268, 1972.

12. M.B. Goldstein, M.F. Pinsky and F.C. Fraser, *Genet. Res. Camb. 4 (2)*, 258, 1963.

13. A.C. Verrusio, D.R. Pollard and F.C. Fraser, *Science 160*, 206, 1968.

14. D.R. Pollard and F.C. Fraser, *Teratology 1*, 335, 1968.

15. R. Goldschmidt, *in* Physiological Genetics, McGraw-Hill, New York, p. 276, ff., 1938.

16. S. Zamenhof, E. van Marthens and L. Gravel, *Science 172*, 850, 1971.

17. W.E. Nance, *in* Nervous System, Birth Defects: Original Article Series VII (1), p. 97, 1971

18. M. Preus and F.C. Fraser, *Clin. Genet. 2*, 331, 1971.

19. P.S. Harper and P.R. Dyken, *Lancet II (7767)*, 53, 1972.

THE USE OF TWIN STUDIES IN THE ANALYSIS OF PHENOTYPIC TRAITS IN MAN[1]

Walter E. Nance[2]
Minoru Nakata[3]
Thomas D. Paul[4]
Pao-lo Yu[5]

The value of twin studies "as a criterion of the relative powers of nature and nurture" has been widely recognized since Galton[1] first introduced the twin study method in 1876. An analysis of the distribution of abnormalities or disease states in twins can provide important clues as to the etiology of the trait in question. However, the study of rare traits in twins can be fraught with serious ascertainment biases[2] that are often difficult to estimate if concordant affected twins are either more or less likely to be reported than discordant twins.

The co-twin control study is a second technique that has probably not been adequately exploited for clinical research.[3] Christian and Kang have shown that for several biochemical traits, observations on identical twins are more than twenty times as efficient as measurements on singletons for detecting significant treatment (environmental) effects.[4] This implies that for these variables, more than 20 times as many unrelated individuals would be required than twins to demonstrate that a constant difference between two groups is

[1]This work was supported by a grant from the John A. Hartford Foundation and was completed during the tenure of a Fogarty International Fellowship to M.N.
[2]Professor of Medical Genetics and Medicine, Indiana University School of Medicine.
[3]Fogarty International Fellow at the Department of Medical Genetics, Indiana University School of Medicine.
[4]Graduate student in Medical Genetics, Indiana University School of Medicine.
[5]Associate Professor of Medical Genetics, Indiana University School of Medicine.

statistically significant.

We are presently involved in two additional types of twin studies. In the first study we are applying the multivariate analytic techniques of Vandenberg[7] to the analysis of interrelated metric traits. In the second study we are exploiting the unique relationship of the offspring of identical twins to separate clearly genetic and environmental influences on metric traits. Analysis of the data will also permit measurement of the additive and dominance components of the genetic variance and may lead to the recognition of human traits that are influenced by heritable factors in the cytoplasm.

Ascertainment of Twins

Twins have been ascertained from multiple sources including (a) consecutive newborn twins at three participating hospitals, (b) social organizations, such as the Mothers of Twins Club, (c) the National Research Council Veterans Twin Panel, and (d) from a review of state vital statistics records. Zygosity is determined by the similarity method and typing of the twins and their parents for more than 20 heritable blood and salivary factors. The present age distribution of twins in the Indiana University Twin Panel is shown in Table 1.

Multivariate Analysis of Correlated Metric Traits

Monozygotic (MZ) twins arise from a single fertilized egg and have identical sets of nuclear genes. Differences between monozygotic twins must therefore arise from environmental factors, discordant somatic mutations and cytoplasmic differences, or from interactions among these factors. It is known that monozygotic twinning may occur at any stage of development up to at least the middle of the second week of embryonic life.[5] Differences in the stage at which twinning occurs are reflected in the marked variation in placentation that is known to occur with MZ twins.[6] MZ twins with two placentae and separate membranes are thought to arise when the twinning process occurs at a very early stage of development, possibly as early as the two-cell stage. In contrast, twins with a single chorion, and especially those with a single amnion, arise at a much later stage by duplication of the inner cell mass or by the induction of two growth centers on the embryonic disc leading to the formation of two primitive streaks. Early and late forming MZ twins can differ substantially in their intra-pair variance, and it is possible that these two classes of MZ twins are epidemiologically distinct. Ideally, MZ twins should be grouped by placental type and tested for heterogeneity, but in practice this is seldom possible with adult twins because the relevant details of the placentation are seldom adequately documented in available medical records.

In contrast, dizygotic (DZ) twins arise from two separate fertilized eggs and may exhibit differences between these factors. Therefore, a comparison of

TABLE 1

Distribution of Twins by Age, Sex and Zygosity

Sex and zygosity class	Age of twins in years						Total
	0–5	6–10	11–15	16–20	21–50	50	
MZ males	7	10	14	8	25	15	79
DZ males	10	5	7	9	33	17	81
MZ females	23	8	11	16	2	2	62
DZ females	14	4	6	3	1	1	29
DZ mixed	33	4	9	7	0	1	54
TOTAL	87	31	47	43	61	36	305

intrapair variances in DZ and MZ twins by means of the F statistic provides a test for the existance of significant genetic determinants of the trait in question, since

$$F = \frac{\sigma^2_{WDZ}}{\sigma^2_{WMZ}} = \frac{\sigma^2_E + \sigma^2_G}{\sigma^2_E}$$

where σ^2_E = the environmental component of the variance, σ^2_G = the genetic component of variance, σ^2_{WDZ} = within pair variance of DZ twins and σ^2_{WMZ} = within pair variance of MZ twins. This test has been widely used for the genetic analysis of individual metric traits in twins. It is assumed that the environmental variances in MZ and DZ twins provides an estimate of the genetic variance in DZ twins.

In 1965, Vandenberg[7] introduced a new multivariate technique for the analysis of interrelated metric traits in twins. Conceptually, the method is an extension of univariate analysis where the intrapair variances of DZ and MZ twins are replaced by co-variance matrices of intrapair differences for multiple variables in the two classes of twins. The method permits the identification of the number of significant independent dimensions of heritable variation that influence the traits along with the particular variables that are influenced by each factor. The method has been described in detail by Bock and Vandenberg,[8] who used the procedure to explore the genetic interrelationship of mental ability subtest scores. We have applied the technique to cephalometric[9] and to dermatoglyphic variables. In both data sets, several of the multivariate genetic factors identified by the analysis were intuitively plausible, a finding which encourages us to believe that this approach may prove to be a useful technique for the analysis of complex genetic traits in man.

Cephalometric Data

Lateral cephalometric roentgenograms were obtained on 24 MZ and 21 like-sexed DZ twin pairs ranging in age from 10 to 17 years. Eight cephalometric measurements were included in the analysis, as shown in Fig. 1, along with stature. The cephalometric variables included six linear and two angular measurements. Univariate analysis showed that genetic factors made a significant contribution to the observed variation in all the traits, with heritability estimates, using Holtzinger formula,[10] ranging from 0.59–0.86 (Table 2).

Table 3 shows the correlation matrix of intrapair differences in MZ twins. Most of the correlations of intrapair differences are small in magnitude and not significantly different from zero. This is an indication that the environmental factors which produce differences in one variable are in general unrelated to factors which produce differences in other variables. An analysis of MZ twins

26

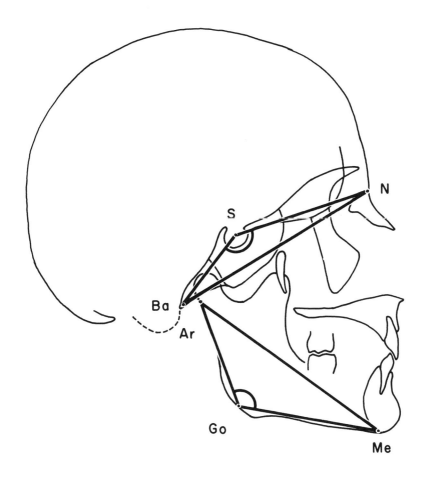

Fig. 1. Diagram of lateral skull x-ray showing six linear and two angular measurements used along with stature in the analysis of cephalometric variables. N: Nasion; S: Sella; Ba: Basion; Ar: Articulare; Go: Gonion; Me: Menton.

TABLE 2

Univariate Analysis of Cephalometric Data in 24
Monozygotic and 21 Like-sexed
Dizygotic Twins

Variable	V_{DZ}/V_{MZ}	$H^2 = \dfrac{V_{DZ} - V_{MZ}}{V_{DZ}}$
1 S–N	3.36**	.70
2 S–Ba	2.91**	.66
3 N–Ba	6.94**	.86
4 Go–Me	2.88**	.65
5 Ar–Go	2.41*	.59
6 Ar–Me	6.21**	.84
7 ∠ N–S–Ba	6.01**	.83
8 ∠ Go	3.31**	.70
9 Stature	3.38**	.70

*p < .05
**p < .01

28

TABLE 3

Correlation Matrix[a] of Intrapair Differences in 24 Monozygotic Twin Pairs:
Cephalometric Data

Variable	S.D.	1	2	3	4	5	6	7	8	9
1 S–N	1.08	1.00								
2 S–Ba	1.43	.11	1.00							
3 N–Ba	1.73	.26	**.58**	1.00						
4 Go–Me	2.00	**.54**	.18	.39	1.00					
5 Ar–Go	2.30	.17	.13	.03	.24	1.00				
6 Ar–Me	2.42	.21	.15	.17	**.61**	**.73**	1.00			
7 ∠ N–S–Ba	1.72	.16	-.28	-.08	.01	.23	.16	1.00		
8 ∠ Go	2.54	**-.47**	-.14	-.14	**-.53**	-.36	-.09	.00	1.00	
9 Stature	.99	.23	-.23	-.16	-.16	.11	.21	**.48**	.05	1.00

Note: Correlations significant at the 5 percent level are shown in bold face type.
[a]Symmetrical elements omitted.

who are discordant for a specific disease state, such as overt diabetes or cancer, could lead to the identification of unexpected phenotypic associations that are caused by a single environmental factor. Similarly, a comparison of the findings in MZ twins with different placental types could lead to the recognition of systematic differences in early and late forming MZ twins. Related measurement errors comprise a final cause for a significant correlation in intrapair differences that must be considered. It seems likely that the apparent correlation between the Articulare-Gonion (Ar—Go) differences and the Articulare-Menton (Ar—Me) differences is an example of this type of measurement error since the length of both line segments depends on the placement of a single point, Ar. In contrast the correlation matrix of intrapair differences in DZ twins (Table 4) has many significant values, a fact which suggests immediately that a few genetic factors influence these variables in a complex manner.

In Table 5, the roots of the determinental equation relating the two co-variance matrices are given. X^2 analysis indicated that there were four significant roots, implying that at least four significant independent dimensions of hereditary variation contribute to the overall variation in the nine measurements. Subject to the constraint that there are only four hereditary factors, the correlation matrix of heritable components was generated from these four significant roots and the matrix of weights of the discriminant functions associated with every root. Many of the variables showed heritable correlations that were greater than 0.7 (Table 6).

In an effort to obtain more insight into the meaning of the results, a rotated factor analysis was performed to identify the major variables that are influenced by each of the four genetic factors. In Table 7, it can be seen that the two horizontal mandibular measurements and stature are the major variables that are influenced by one factor. A second factor influenced the horizontal cranial base measurements along with mandibular gonial angle. A third factor influenced the cranial base angle, and finally the fourth factor affected the posterior cranial base and the mandibular ramus along with stature.

It has been found from multivariate analysis of cephalometric data from unrelated individuals[11] and from experimental cross-mating studies in dogs[12] that the upper and lower jaws appear to have independent determinants, which may well be genetic, and are thought to play a role in the etiology of malocclusion. It is possible that the independence of the first two factors identified in this study can be considered to imply a separate genetic determination of these two parts of the cranio-facial complex, although the variables selected for the present analysis were not ideally suited to demonstrate this fact.

The last factor, which is composed of the posterior cranial base, the ramus

TABLE 4

Correlation Matrix[a] of Intrapair Differences in 21 Pairs of Like-sexed Dizygotic Twins: Cephalometric Data

Variable	S.D.	1	2	3	4	5	6	7	8	9
1 S–N	1.97	1.00								
2 S–Ba	2.45	**.48**	1.00							
3 N–Ba	4.60	**.75**	**.77**	1.00						
4 Go–Me	3.40	**.52**	.42	.41	1.00					
5 Ar–Go	3.57	.16	**.57**	.34	.41	1.00				
6 Ar–Me	6.04	.44	**.55**	**.57**	**.76**	**.65**	1.00			
7 ∠ N–S–Ba	4.21	-.08	.06	.36	-.02	-.09	.24	1.00		
8 ∠ Go	4.62	.12	.03	.33	**-.45**	-.13	.06	**.45**	1.00	
9 Stature	1.82	.36	**.49**	.30	**.46**	.32	**.49**	-.29	-.15	1.00

Note: Correlations significant at the 5 percent level are shown in bold face type.
[a]Symmetrical elements omitted.

31

TABLE 5

Transformation Matrix of Heritable Variation in Cephalometric Variables Showing Discriminant Functions for Each Root Along with Eigen Values, Chi-square Tests, P Values and Intra Class Correlation Coefficients

Variable	1	2	3	4	5	6	7	8	9
1 S–N	-.22	.07	.56	.74	-.01	-.05	-.05	-.45	.58
2 S–Ba	.06	.02	-.08	-.46	-.08	.15	.23	.73	.07
3 N–Ba	-.31	.03	.41	-.04	-.24	-.17	-.26	-.42	-.27
4 Go–Me	1.90	.26	.07	-.31	.29	-.39	.87	-.08	-.12
5 Ar–Go	1.69	.09	.42	-.35	.30	-.15	.11	-.16	.13
6 Ar–Me	-2.08	-.19	-.30	.30	.07	.18	-.40	-.10	-.03
7 ∠ N–S–Ba	-.09	.59	-.22	-.20	-.10	-.00	.10	.02	.21
8 ∠ Go	1.11	.27	.39	-.04	.27	.08	.41	.01	-.05
9 Stature	-.19	.87	.28	-.39	-.38	-.36	.28	-.39	.17
Eigen values	36.2	13.6	11.0	3.7	2.4	1.7	.9	.6	.2
Chi-square	391.0	288.1	212.5	142.6	99.6	66.0	38.1	20.3	6.7
Degrees of freedom	189.	160	133	108	85	64	45	28	13
P	<.0005	<.0005	<.0005	<.025	<.05	<.05	<.05	<.05	<.05
r_i	.97	.92	.90	.73	.58	.44	.0	0	0

TABLE 6

Correlation Matrix[a] of Heritable Variation of Cephalometric Data

Variable	S.D.	1	2	3	4	5	6	7	8	9
1 S–N	1.65	1.00								
2 S–Ba	2.06	.55	1.00							
3 N–Ba	4.18	**.79**	**.82**	1.00						
4 Go–Me	2.32	.44	.55	.42	1.00					
5 Ar–Go	2.28	.30	**.92**	.56	.43	1.00				
6 Ar–Me	5.03	.58	**.74**	**.74**	**.90**	.53	1.00			
7 ∠N–S–Ba	3.94	-.06	.11	.40	.01	-.11	.31	1.00		
8 ∠Go	3.45	.51	.21	.67	-.27	-.06	.11	.57	1.00	
9 Stature	1.57	.51	**.70**	.39	**.82**	**.71**	**.70**	.21	.37	1.00

Note: Correlations of .70 or more are shown in bold faced type.
[a]Symmetrical elements omitted.

TABLE 7

Related Factor Analysis of Heritable Components in Cephalometric Data

Variable	Factor loadings				Total
	1	2	3	4	
1 S–N	37	**89**	19	15	
2 S–Ba	36	33	- 07	**86**	
3 N–Ba	30	**73**	- 32	50	
4 Go–Me	**97**	04	03	21	
5 Ar–Go	22	04	10	**96**	
6 Ar–Me	**84**	28	- 24	36	
7 ∠N–S–Ba	05	11	**99**	- 02	
8 ∠Go	-30	**80**	- 50	01	
9 Stature	**71**	08	46	**51**	
Total proportion of heritable variance	29.4	24.2	18.4	26.3	98.3
Variance accounted for by variables shown in bold type	23.9	21.8	10.9	21.3	77.9

34

of the mandible and stature, is readily interpretable. The spheno-occipital synchondrosis, which is measured in variable S–Ba, and the condylar cartilage of the mandible, which is reflected in the variable Ar–Go, have cartilaginous elements[13,14] and resemble the long bones of the axial skeleton in their epiphyseal growth pattern rather than the membranous bones that make up most of the remainder of the skull. The axial skeleton, of course, makes a major contribution to overall stature.

It would clearly be an oversimplification to equate the genetic factors identified in this analysis with single gene effects. However, in the case of the first factor, single gene mutations are known which profoundly affect the development of the lower jaw.[15,16] Similarly, in the case of the last factor, monogenic traits, such as classical achondroplasia, are known which have a dramatic effect on both the overall stature and the length of the cranial base. We know of no published analysis of mandibular measurements in achondro- plastic dwarfs, but predict that the mandibular ramus would likewise be small in comparison with dimensions involving the membranous bones of the skull.

Dermatoglyphic Data

Palmar and digital dermatoglyphics were available on 80 MZ and 45 like- sexed DZ twin pairs. Sixteen variables were studied including ridge counts for each of the 10 digits (variables 7–16 in Table 8), left and right atd angle and right proximal and distal triradial measurements. As might be expected (Table 9), there were significant correlations in the intrapair differences in MZ twins for the proximal and distal triradial measurements and the atd angles in each hand. The remaining significant correlations are few in number and gen- erally small in magnitude. In contrast, there are a large number of significant correlations between intrapair differences among the DZ twins (Table 10). Eight of the 16 roots of the determinantal equation relating the MZ and DZ co-variance matrices were significant by the X^2 test (Table 11). Table 12 shows the correlation matrix of heritable components calculated under the assumption that only eight independent hereditary factors influence the 16 variables. Twenty-three of the 120 correlations were .70 or more, and high correlations were particularly numerous among the ridge count variables. The rotated factor loadings are shown in Table 13. The pattern that emerges is striking. Whatever the genetic factors are that influence the ridge count on the left little finger, they also appear to influence the right little finger (Factor II). Similarly, a separate factor (III) has a major influence on the ridge count of both thumbs while most of the middle fingers of both hands are influenced by yet another factor. Independent factors appear to influence the two triradial measurements but, interestingly, there is evidence for separate determination of

TABLE 8

Univariate Analysis of Dermatoglyphic Data in 80 Monozygotic and 45 Like-sexed Dizygotic Twins

	Variable	V_{DZ}/V_{MZ}	$H^2 = \dfrac{V_{DZ}-V_{MZ}}{V_{DZ}}$
1	Proximal left triradial measurement (L–Pt)	2.43**	.58
2	Distal left triradial measurement (L–Dt)	2.52**	.60
3	Proximal right triradial measurement (R–Pt)	1.67*	.40
4	Distal right triradial measurement (R–Dt)	2.16**	.53
5	Left atd angle (L–atd)	2.74**	.63
6	Right atd angle (R–atd)	2.87**	.65
7	Ridge count, left thumb (L–T)	3.92**	.74
8	Ridge count, left index finger (L–2)	4.06**	.75
9	Ridge count, left 3rd finger (L–3)	5.02**	.80
10	Ridge count, left 4th finger (L–4)	4.18**	.76
11	Ridge count, left 5th finger (L–5)	3.44**	.70
12	Ridge count, right thumb (R–T)	3.26**	.69
13	Ridge count, right index finger (R–2)	2.70**	.62
14	Ridge count, right 3rd finger (R–3)	4.75**	.78
15	Ridge count, right 4th finger (R–4)	4.72**	.78
16	Ridge count, right 5th finger (R–5)	3.09**	.67

*p < .05
**p < .01

TABLE 9

Correlation Matrix[a] of Intrapair Differences in 80 Monozygotic Twin Pairs: Dermatoglyphic Data

	Variable	S.D.	1	2	3	4	5	6	7	8	9	10	11	12	13	14	15	16
1	L–Pt	.54	1.00															
2	L–Dt	.27	**.35**	1.00														
3	R–Pt	.59	.20	.05	1.00													
4	R–Dt	.30	.02	**.26**	**.36**	1.00												
5	L–atd	4.30	**.74**	.05	.16	-.10	1.00											
6	R–atd	4.69	.14	-.06	**.61**	.14	.20	1.00										
7	L–T	2.09	.12	**.27**	.15	.20	.11	-.02	1.00									
8	L–2	2.86	-.21	-.08	-.13	-.04	-.15	-.07	-.05	1.00								
9	L–3	2.36	-.14	-**.26**	-.05	-.07	-.01	-.05	-.02	**.26**	1.00							
10	L–4	2.57	.08	-.01	**.25**	.12	.06	.18	.12	-.12	.18	1.00						
11	L–5	2.05	.00	-.06	-.08	-.04	.02	-.09	.14	.10	.17	.04	1.00					
12	R–T	2.15	-.01	.00	.03	.09	-.04	.08	-.01	.19	-.16	-.08	-.18	1.00				
13	R–2	3.07	-.06	.10	-.13	.12	-.11	.08	.03	.07	-.02	-.04	.00	.14	1.00			
14	R–3	2.02	.03	.11	.02	-.01	-.06	-.08	-.08	.03	.01	.19	-.19	-.09	.15	1.00		
15	R–4	2.28	-.10	-.11	.15	-.03	.02	-.07	.06	.20	-.05	**.26**	-.01	.11	.17	**.25**	1.00	
16	R–5	2.16	-.05	-.19	.00	-.01	.05	-.04	-.08	.10	-.08	.03	.00	.09	-.07	.10	.18	1.00

Note: Correlations significant at the 5 percent level are shown in bold face type.
[a]Symmetrical elements omitted.

TABLE 10

Correlation Matrix[a] of Intrapair Differences in 45 Pairs of Like-sexed Dizygotic Twins : Dermatoglyphic Data

Variance	S.D.	1	2	3	4	5	6	7	8	9	10	11	12	13	14	15	16
1 L-Pt	.84	1.00															
2 L-Dt	.43	**.31**	1.00														
3 R-Pt	.76	**.58**	.15	1.00													
4 R-Dt	.44	.11	**.73**	.24	1.00												
5 L-atd	7.13	**.53**	.02	**.32**	.03	1.00											
6 R-atd	7.95	**.32**	.02	**.60**	.00	.08	1.00										
7 L-T	4.14	.15	.01	-.22	.07	.24	.08	1.00									
8 L-2	5.77	.07	.00	.13	.00	-.18	.23	.46	1.00								
9 L-3	5.29	.02	-.16	-.07	.08	-.02	.34	.47	.60	1.00							
10 L-4	5.25	-.09	.00	-.13	-.03	-.22	.06	.43	.61	.61	1.00						
11 L-5	3.80	-.09	-.05	.05	.04	-.17	.26	.40	.52	.57	.58	1.00					
12 R-T	3.87	-.14	.05	.32	.04	-.18	.11	.70	.39	.51	.47	.32	1.00				
13 R-2	5.05	-.03	-.12	-.04	.02	-.16	.32	.28	.65	.69	.52	.49	.46	1.00			
14 R-3	4.41	-.02	.17	-.03	.09	-.03	.20	.39	.53	.76	.59	.40	.48	.75	1.00		
15 R-4	4.95	-.14	.17	-.13	.02	-.22	.10	.43	.49	.63	.66	.47	.47	.47	.62	1.00	
16 R-5	3.79	.00	.00	-.06	-.10	.00	.14	.32	.52	.48	.57	.70	.23	.44	.36	.57	1.00

Note: Correlations significant at the 5 percent level are shown in bold face type.
[a] Symmetrical elements omitted.

38

TABLE 11

Eigen Values of MZ–DZ Discriminant Functions for Dermatoglyphic Data Along with Chi-square Tests and P values

	1	2	3	4	5	6	7	8	9 ... 10
Variances	21.6	7.1	6.6	5.6	4.1	2.8	2.3	2.2	Omitted from Table
Chi-square	1346.9	1104.5	953.3	807.6	673.3	559.9	470.7	392.3	
Degrees of freedom	720	660	602	546	492	440	390	342	
P	<.0005	<.0005	<.0005	<.0005	<.0005	<.005	<.005	<.05	<.05 ...

39

TABLE 12
Correlation Matrix[a] of Heritable Variation of Dermatoglyphic Data

Variation	S.D.	1	2	3	4	5	6	7	8	9	10	11	12	13	14	15	16
1 L–Pt	.60	1.00															
2 L–Dt	.35	.39	1.00														
3 R–Pt	.52	**.85**	.23	1.00													
4 R–Dt	.34	.24	**.90**	.15	1.00												
5 L–atd	4.87	.26	.09	.38	.21	1.00											
6 R–atd	6.36	.43	.07	.63	-.05	-.01	1.00										
7 L–T	3.59	-.34	-.06	-.49	.02	-.53	.14	1.00									
8 L–2	5.11	-.06	.02	-.14	-.01	-.28	.35	.57	1.00								
9 L–3	4.79	.04	.29	-.05	.15	-.07	.49	.60	**.70**	1.00							
10 L–4	4.61	-.16	.02	-.36	-.08	-.38	.01	.58	**.80**	**.72**	1.00						
11 L–5	3.28	-.08	.01	.04	.02	-.24	.38	.51	.64	.68	**.74**	1.00					
12 R–T	3.27	-.30	.02	-.51	.04	-.36	.09	**.94**	.50	**.72**	.62	.47	1.00				
13 R–2	4.14	.15	.10	.08	-.01	.01	.54	.49	**.84**	**.92**	**.76**	**.71**	.57	1.00			
14 R–3	3.85	.06	.20	-.10	.08	.10	.34	.53	.67	**.96**	**.72**	.57	**.71**	**.92**	1.00		
15 R–4	4.33	-.22	.30	-.35	.06	-.44	.18	.52	.56	**.81**	**.78**	.61	.63	.65	**.72**	1.00	
16 R–5	3.09	-.15	.03	-.05	-.04	-.26	.29	.38	.69	.68	**.82**	**.95**	.37	**.77**	.59	**.72**	1.00

Note: Correlations of .70 or more are shown in bold face type

[a] Symmetrical elements omitted.

40

TABLE 13

Rotated Factor Analysis of Heritable Components in Dermatoglyphic Data

Variable		Factor Loadings								Total
		1	2	3	4	5	6	7	8	
1	L–Pt	-.05	.11	.13	.19	**.95**	.06	.11	-.01	
2	L–Dt	.22	.04	.09	**.94**	-.19	.07	.00	.06	
3	R–Pt	-.15	-.10	.29	.10	-.78	-.21	.46	.06	
4	R–Dt	.05	-.02	-.09	**.98**	-.05	.14	-.02	.03	
5	L–atd	.03	.13	.24	.09	-.13	**.94**	.00	.07	
6	R–atd	-.23	-.14	-.06	-.04	-.36	.03	**.88**	.09	
7	L–T	.27	-.19	**.85**	.00	.22	.27	.06	.18	
8	L–2	.47	-.37	-.20	-.01	.02	.14	.12	**.74**	
9	L–3	**.82**	-.32	-.33	-.16	-.01	.01	.24	.12	
10	L–4	**.62**	-.55	-.20	-.06	-.05	.24	.29	.34	
11	L–5	.31	**.90**	.24	.00	-.01	.06	.15	.09	
12	R–T	.50	-.12	**.81**	.02	.20	.13	.03	-.02	
13	R–2	**.75**	-.39	-.22	-.03	-.15	.11	.22	.37	
14	R–3	**.87**	-.23	-.32	.06	-.04	.18	.06	-.17	
15	R–4	**.79**	-.35	-.09	.16	.23	-.40	.02	.04	
16	R–5	.43	**.86**	.00	-.01	.08	.13	.08	-.16	
Total proportion of heritable variance		24.9	16.0	12.5	12.3	11.8	8.6	7.8	6.0	99.9
Variance accounted for by variables shown in bold type		18.7	9.6	8.6	11.5	9.4	5.5	4.8	3.4	71.5

41

of the atd angles. We regard the extent to which homologous measurements on the two hands were grouped together as a rather remarkable confirmation of the ability of this technique to pick out biologically meaningful relationships between correlated metric traits.

Our experience in these two studies suggests that it may often be possible to find valid and useful interpretations for the genetic factors identified by multivariate analysis of twin data. Furthermore, the technique may also provide a new approach to the study of birth defects. By looking for specific sets of genetically determined phenotypic correlations in normal twins, it is possible that we might be able to infer whether the multiple phenotypic features of an idiopathic congenital malformation syndrome such as the Taybi-Rubenstein syndrome[17] or the Cornelia DeLange syndrome,[18] for example, have a multifactorial or chromosomal basis or whether they are the pleotropic manifestations of mutant genes at a single locus.

Genetic Study of Human Half-sibs

Genetic analysis of half-sib data has long been recognized to be one of the most effective available techniques for separating genetic and environmental effects.[19] In conjunction with full-sib and parent-offspring correlations, half-sib data permit a partitioning of the total genetic variance into its additive and dominance components. The contribution of epistatic interactions between additive genes can even be estimated from half-sib data[20] as well as the effects of X-linked genes and maternal factors.

Despite the great potential of the method, half-sib studies have not been widely exploited in human genetics research. In contrast to experimental organisms, human matings cannot, in general, be planned by the investigator; and since monogamy, or at most sequential polygamy, is the most prevalent mating pattern in many contemporary societies, the opportunities for conventional half-sib studies in man are somewhat limited. Furthermore, conventional half-sibs are seldom the same age, and the physical and psychological environments to which they are exposed vary widely from family to family and are extremely difficult to characterize in many cases even in the most general terms, such as "normal", "similar" or "different". Finally, in the case of half-sibs resulting from illegitimacy, death of the husband or wife, or divorce, all of the relevant parents are seldom available for study.

The offspring of identical twins would appear to constitute a unique class of human half-sibs in which most of these methodologic difficulties can be circumvented. Since they are ascertained through parents of the same age and sex, MZ twin half-sibships would have the same expected size and mean age. In general, these children experience a home environment which is no different from the families of singletons. Finally, in contrast to conventional half-sibs,

42

all of the parents are usually eager to cooperate.

Some of the parameters that may be estimated from the genetic relationships in the families of monozygotic twins are shown in Table 14. These parameters may be used to measure several important variance components.

Environmental Variance

Several informative estimates and comparisons of environmental variance emerge from the analysis. The within pair variance of MZ twins provides a traditional estimate of the influence on the trait in question and of environmental differences between twins. However, this variance component includes factors that are unique to monozygotic twins such as placental differences and certain perinatal hazards not shared by singletons. It will be instructive to compare this variance component with the between spouse co-variance. The latter may be resolved into two components: between and within MZ pairs. If assortative mating has a significant influence on the trait in question, it will inflate the between pair component of variance, V_{EC}; in this case, the within pair component, V_{EW}, may provide a more valid measure of environmental effects.

The existence of maternal effects on the trait in question may be sought by a comparison of full-sibships within paternal and maternal half-sibships. A comparison of the offspring-aunt and the offspring-uncle co-variances will provide a second test for the existence of a significant maternal effect and/or differences in the similarities of the home environment (diet, socioeconomic status, education, etc.) provided by monozygotic females as opposed to monozygotic males.

These comparisons should permit the selection of appropriate values of V_{EC} and V_{EW} to be used for estimation of the additive and dominance components of the genetic variance.

Dominance Deviations

The variance component attributable to dominance may be estimated from the between half-sibship co-variance and the between sibship (within half-sibship) co-variance after appropriate adjustment for possible differences in the environmental components of the two co-variances. If there is no evidence for epistatic interactions between additive genes (see below), the extent to which the latter exceeds the former will estimate one-fourth of the dominance component of variance. A second estimate may be derived from a comparison of the full-sib co-variance and the parent offspring co-variance, after appropriate corrections for additive epistasis.

Additive Genetic Variance

Half-sib studies provide a unique opportunity to measure the additive

TABLE 14
Variance Components of Genetic Relationships in the Families of Monozygotic Twins

Relationship	Parameter	Variance Components		
		Additive $V_A + V_{AA} + ...$	Dominance V_D	Environment $V_{EC} + V_{EW}$
Between MZ twin pairs	σ^2_{BMZ}	$V_A + V_{AA} + ...$	V_D	V_{EC}
Within MZ twin pairs	σ^2_{WMZ}			V_{EW}
Between half-sibships	cov HS	$1/4\,V_A + 1/16\,V_{AA} + ...$		V_{EC}
Maternal half-fraternities	cov HS_M	$1/4\,V_A + 1/16\,V_{AA} + ...$		V_{ECM}
Paternal half-fraternities	cov HS_P	$1/4\,V_A + 1/16\,V_{AA} + ...$		V_{ECP}
Between full sibships within HS	cov FS - cov HS	$1/4\,V_A + 3/16\,V_{AA} + ...$	$1/4\,V_D$	V'_{EC}
Maternal HS	cov FS_M - cov HS_M	$1/4\,V_A + 3/16\,V_{AA} + ...$	$1/4\,V_D$	V'_{ECM}
Paternal HS	cov FS_P - cov HS_P	$1/4\,V_A + 3/16\,V_{AA} + ...$	$1/4\,V_D$	V'_{ECP}
Within full sibships	V_P - cov FS	$1/2\,V_A + 1/4\,V_{AA} + ...$	$3/4\,V_D$	V_{EW}
Between spouse	cov SP			$V'_{EC} + V'_{EW}$
Between MZ pairs	cov SP_B			V'_{EC}
Within MZ pairs	cov $\overline{SP_W}$			V'_{EW}
Mid-parent offspring	cov $\overline{OP}$	$1/2\,V_A + 1/4\,V_{AA} + ...$		V_{EC}
Twin parent offspring	cov OP	$1/2\,V_A + 1/4\,V_{AA} + ...$		V_{EC}
Maternal twin	cov OP_M	$1/2\,V_A + 1/4\,V_{AA} + ...$		V_{ECM}
Paternal twin	cov OP_P	$1/2\,V_A + 1/4\,V_{AA} + ...$		V_{ECP}
Offspring-twin aunt or uncle	cov OAU	$1/2\,V_A + 1/4\,V_{AA} + ...$		V'_{EC}
Aunt	cov OA	$1/2\,V_A + 1/4\,V_{AA} + ...$		V'_{ECM}
Uncle	cov OU	$1/2\,V_A + 1/4\,V_{AA} + ...$		V'_{ECP}

component of the genetic variance from observations made on members of the same generation, since the co-variance of half-sibs, suitably corrected for environmental variance, estimates ¼ V_A. A comparison of maternal and paternal half-fraternities would provide an estimate of the contribution of additive genes on the X-chromosome to the overall effect. If differences are found, it should be possible to exclude environmental factors as a cause for the observed effects by appropriate comparisons between maternal and paternal half-sibships and maternal and paternal half-sororities. A comparison of the estimates of additive variance derived from the half-sib data with that derived from the parent offspring co-variance will provide a unique opportunity to measure epistatic interactions between additive loci since these interactions make at least twice as great a contribution to the parent-offspring co-variance as they do to the half-sib co-variance. Epistatic interactions could make an important contribution to many medically significant quantitative traits. We know of no other practical method by which these interactions can be estimated in man.

Many traits that are of interest to human geneticists not only vary with age but have also changed systematically from one generation to the next. A comparison of the two estimates of additive inheritance, one derived from parent-offspring data and the other derived entirely from subjects in the offspring generation may provide an indication of whether the systematic trends have been accompanied by changes in the genetic variance components. For example, it is generally agreed that the striking changes in stature that have occurred in Western societies during the past century are largely attributable to environmental factors or to genetic-environmental interactions rather than genetic selection. The finding that there has been no demonstrable "exhaustion" of the additive variance in the offspring generation would be consistent with this hypothesis.

We recognize that our model does not include many potentially important variance components such as the interaction components between environment and the additive dominance components of the genetic variance. For simplicity, we have included only those components which can be resolved by an analysis of the families of identical twins.

Cytoplasmic Effects

In 1968, Storrs and Williams[21] reported the existence of striking morphologic and biochemical discordances among monozygotic armadillo quadruplets. Since these animals possess identical sets of nuclear genes, the authors reasoned that some of the differences they observed may have arisen from the discordant expression of heritable factors in the cytoplasm. There are, of course, many possible explanations for discordance in newborn MZ twins including somatic mutation, placental differences and a variety of perinatal factors. However, if heritable cytoplasmic differences do make a contribution to intrapair differences in MZ twins, an analysis of the families of identical twins should permit the identification of those traits which are influenced by heritable cytoplasmic factors. In the case of female MZ twins, the direction and magnitude of the intrapair difference in the twin parents should be correlated with the mean difference between their half-sib offspring if the trait is determined by heritable cytoplasmic factors. Male MZ twins may show similar intrapair differences but they should be uncorrelated with the mean differences of their half-sib offspring if the trait in question is influenced by heritable cytoplasmic factors.

We have just begun to study MZ twin half-sibships, and cannot yet provide a numerical example of the foregoing analysis. However, the form that the data will take is illustrated by Fig. 2, which shows the total ridge counts of the first two complete families that we have studied. Note that there is variation between kindred means and within sibships. The ridge counts of MZ twins are remarkably close (but in the case of one husband-wife pair they were identical!) and the sibship means, in general, fall between the values of the parents.

Relevance to Congenital Malformations

The genetic model developed here should be of great value in the further genetic analysis of a variety of medically significant quantitative traits such as serum lipids and other biochemical measurements, blood pressure, glucose tolerance, birthweight, intelligence, pigmentation, dermatoglyphic ridge counts, etc. However, the model has equal relevance to the study of qualitative traits such as birth defects. It is widely believed that several important groups of congenital malformations including cleft lip and palate, midline neurologic defects and pyloric stenosis are determined by multifactorial inheritance with a continuously distributed underlying liability and a discrete developmental threshold for expression of the trait.[22] Three generation data will doubtless provide a critical test of these models for traits that do not interfere greatly with normal reproduction. However, for traits such as midline neurologic defects, an assessment of the observed risk in first and second degree relatives in comparison with the predicted risk has, heretofore, been the only available method for testing the hypothesis. Estimation of the incidence of malformations in the MZ twin half-sibs of affected probands would not only provide a comparison of observed and expected risk in another class of relatives but would also yield critical evidence on the potential significance of maternal and/or cytoplasmic factors in the etiology of the malformations. It might be objected that identical twins are so rare that data of this type would

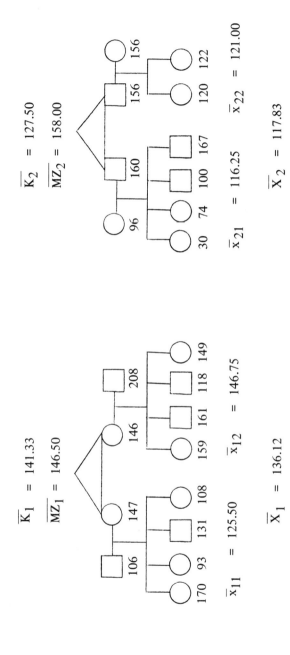

Fig. 2. Pedigrees of two monozygotic twin half-sibships showing individual total ridge counts. Kindred means ($\overline{K}$), sibship means ($\overline{x}$), half-sibship means ($\overline{X}$) and twin pair means ($\overline{MZ}$).

47

be extremely hard to collect. However, in situations where record linkage is feasible, no class of human relatives should be easier to link than identical twins. Fertile monozygotic twins are always of the same sex, and are almost invariably born on the same day and in the same place. Identical twins also have the same surname, of course, and more often than not, they even have names that rhyme!

REFERENCES

1. F. Galton, *J. Anthrop. Inst. Grt. Brit. and Ireland 5,* 291, 1876.

2. G. Allen, *Prog. in Med. Genet. 4,* 242, 1965.

3. W.E. Nance, *Medicine 38,* 403, 1959.

4. J.C. Christian and K.W. Kang, *Metabolism 21,* 291, 1972.

5. M.G. Bulmer, *in* The Biology of Twinning in Man, Clarendon Press, Oxford, pp. 25–45, 1970.

6. S.J. Strong and G. Corney, *in* The Placenta in Twin Pregnancy, Pergamon Press, London, pp. 1–134, 1967.

7. S.G. Vandenberg (Ed.), *in* Methods and Goals in Human Behavior Genetics, Academic Press, New York, pp. 29–43, 1965.

8. R.D. Bock and S.G. Vandenberg, *in* Progress in Human Behavior Genetics, S.G. Vandenberg (Ed.), Johns Hopkins Press, Baltimore, pp. 233–260, 1968.

9. M. Nakata, P. Yu, B. Davis and W.E. Nance, *Amer. J. Hum. Genet.,* in press.

10. K.J. Holzinger, *J. Educ. Psychol. 20,* 241, 1940.

11. B. Solow, *Amer. Odont. Scand. 46,* 1, 1966.

12. A.L. Johnson, *Amer. J. Orthodont. 26,* 627, 1940.

13. T.M. Graber, *in* Orthodontics, 2nd Ed.,W.B. Saunders Co., Philadelphia, pp. 47–51, 1966.

14. H. Sicher, *in* Oral Anatomy, 3rd Ed., C.V. Mosby, St. Louis, pp. 99–134, 1960.

15. D. Bixler and J.S. Christian, *Birth Defects Orig. Art. Ser. 7,* 67, 1971.

16. S. Pruzansky, *Birth Defects Orig. Art. Ser. V (2),* 120, 1969.

17. J.H. Rubenstein, *Birth Defects Orig. Art. Ser. V (2),* 25, 1969.

18. D.W. Smith, *in* Recognizable Patterns of Human Malformation, W.B. Saunders, Philadelphia, pp. 62–63, 1970.

19. D.S. Falconer, *in* Introduction to Quantitative Genetics, Oliver and Boyd, Edinburgh, pp. 150–164, 1960.

20. R.E. Comstock, *Cold Spring Harbor Symp. Quant. Biol. 20,* 93, 1965.

21. E.E. Storrs and R.J. Williams, *Proc. Nat. Acad. Sci. 60,* 910, 1968.

22. C.O. Carter, *Prog. Med. Genet 4,* 59, 1965.

DISCUSSION

DR. HOOK: Dr. Neel, some years ago you and Dr. Bloom reported an increased frequency of chromosome breaks in individuals from this primitive society. Is this a reflection of increased mutagens in the environment and might it provide some direct evidence for environmental teratogens as well, consistent with the observations of birth defects in this group?

DR. NEEL: Yes, we did find a surprisingly high frequency of chromosomal breakage in one Indian village. We thought we would find a record low for chromosome damage in these clean living Indians. Instead, we ran into a record high. This finding came during the first year of the studies, and that was when we published a preliminary paper. We did two further studies. During the second year, we could not confirm the original findings in other villages, so in the third year, we went back to the same villages in which we had found the increased damage but we found no increase. The findings from the first year are quite unequivocal. There is no doubt about the validity of our observations. We can only conclude that some agent, unidentified, hit that village shortly before we came along, producing chromosomal damage, which has now largely disappeared. We have considered aflatoxins and the other kinds of things that you find in nature.

DR. FRASER: Could this be caused by viruses which were brought in?

DR. NEEL: No, not viruses brought in by an invading group, but the Indians, of course, have their own viruses and we have extensive antibody studies to show just how many and how varied these all are. So, considering Dr. Hook's question again — yes, there could well be some teratogenic agent which produces chromosomal damage and this *could* be a cause of congenital defect. We simply don't know.

DR. SKALKO: In respect to the possibility of dietary differences, I would like to know if Dr. Fraser has any ideas or comments on an alternative for the dietary difference such as changes in oogenesis or some other parameter in the strains that he is dealing with.

DR. FRASER: We picked the mitochondria because they are transmitted through the egg cytoplasm and because the NAD analog does inhibit oxidative phosphorylation in the mitochondria. So it seems a logical guess but I don't think we've ruled out viruses. For instance, there are cytoplasmically transmitted viruses that will influence the activity of enzymes. I am not sticking by the mitochondria as the only possible explanation. The field is wide open.

LAWRENCE SHAPIRO (Letchworth Village, Theills, New York): I would like to ask Dr. Nance about the validity of using ridge counts as part of your model. I don't disagree with the heritability of ridge counts but I think it is a complex situation affected by many things — the *in utero* environment, by the development of infection of other maternal agents — and I think that many of the syndromes we see have a significant lowering of ridge counts due to factors that we really don't understand. If you believe what Drs. Mulvahill and Smith have said, the ridge counts and patterns are not inherited, they're really a factor that relates to what's going on in the *in utero* environment at the time that the patterns are being formed. Or they may be related to the shape of the hand which may be inherited. An example which I have seen, was in a pair of monozygotic twins who were discordant for Down's syndrome as a result of mitotic nondysjunction resulting in mosaicism in the twin with Down's syndrome and the normal twin had a finger ridge pattern similar to the parents and other siblings whereas the twin with Down's syndrome had a dermatoglyphic pattern typical of Down's syndrome.

DR. NANCE: I certainly agree that chromosomal abnormalities, and single gene mutations for which monozygotic twins could be discordant (if you assume that this is a somatic event) can profoundly influence the ridge counts. On the other hand, I've always regarded the genetic analysis of ridge counts to be far and away the best model we have in human genetics, of a polygenic or multifactorial trait that really obeys the predictions of the model. So, we use this in our analysis of normal twins to see whether we can dissect out some of the factors and try to ascertain how many independent factors there are that influence the total ridge count.

EMMA K. HARROD (Erie County Department of Health, Buffalo, New York): Could there have been any other causes of high incidences of murmurs in these Indians, such as iron deficiency anemias?

DR. NEEL: These were not the murmurs of iron deficiency anemia. They were harsh organic murmurs. Incidentally, we've done a fair number of hemoglobins and we found some iron deficiency anemia, but not a great deal.

ROSALIE GREEN (Arlington Hospital, Arlington, Virginia): Dr. Neel, has there been a significant degree of inbreeding among these tribes and would you comment on the possibility of a founder effect?

DR. NEEL: There is inbreeding and there are some studies which show that the frequency of congenital defects is higher in the children of cousin marriages than in the children of non-cousin marriages. If we put that together with the possibility that a few of the progenitors of this particular group brought in whatever the genetic basis for congenital heart disease is, yes, we could have a founder effect.

CHESTER A. SWINYARD (Institute of Rehabilitation, New York University Medical Center, New York, New York): I am continuously intrigued by the incidence we get by external examination and the increase by autopsies. In the course of watching the dissection of some 500 human cadavers, I am impressed by variability. The line between variation and malformation is fuzzy. I can't recall that I ever saw a cadaver that didn't have at least one at risk factor. We usually don't call it a malformation.

DR. NEEL: I completely agree with your comments. We always attempt, usually successfully, but sometimes we lose the battle with the editor, to list that which we saw and called a congenital malformation and we have attempted to distinguish between minor and major defects and to present them in separate tables.

DR. SWINYARD: There is a great difference between dissection and autopsy. A dissection will reveal much more than an autopsy, which usually is a rather superficial procedure.

DR. HOOK: This question comes up even at the experimental level. It is really the question of deciding what is a morphologic variation and what is, in fact, a defect. This was recently an issue in an experimental study where the investigators found an increase in morphologic variation but they claimed that what they were looking at was not teratogenic because these were just variants, not defects. Dr. Fraser, would you comment on this?

DR. FRASER: I really don't think that *Science (176,* 262, 1972) was fair to the investigator. If I'm reading you right, 2,4,5,T and its contaminant dioxin, which was said to produce subcutaneous hematomas and edema in offspring of mothers exposed to the teratogens, I think I would agree that one doesn't usually call these malformations. But they are evidence of damage to the embryo and, therefore, just as important as malformations if you are worried about protecting the population. Whether you want to call them teratogens or simply toxic agents, is a matter of taste.

PHILIP BANISTER (Department of National Health and Welfare, Ottawa, Ontario, Canada): Dr. Neel said that he always described the malformation he has seen but then he went on to talk about major malformations. That which is major to me may not be major to you. My plea is that we record the malformations as accurately as possible. I just got the results on a cohort of about 97,000 children born in 1970 that have been followed for a year. I could add them up and say that the total malformation rate was about 4.9%. But, again, we should record the individual anomalies and not lump minor and major malformations together.

BERNARD A. BECKER (University of Iowa, College of Medicine, Iowa City, Iowa): Dr. Fraser is reluctant to get into the discussion of whether effects are teratogenic or embryotoxic. I'm not. It's an important distinction that has to be made by people who are concerned with the effects of chemical substances on developing organisms. The main distinction is that a teratogenic change is a defect in formation. It is a "misbildung", as the Germans put it, on the elaboration of the structure or system. On the other hand, organisms *in utero* are as susceptible to toxic effects or drugs as those which are post-natal. Consequently, it is feasible and realistic to consider toxic effects on developing organisms as separate from teratogenic effects.

DR. FRASER: I thoroughly agree. It was not timidity which kept me out of this argument. From the point of view of people who are worried about the public health effects, they are both bad.

DR. NANCE: Dr. Neel, would you comment on the relationship of inbreeding to the phenodeviant hypothesis? You said you were struck by the fact that most populations have the same overall incidence of malformations. Is this what you would expect in populations that vary in their inbreeding coefficient, or not?

DR. NEEL: Most populations do not vary enough in their inbreeding coefficient that this approach is a good test of the phenodeviant hypothesis. This hypothesis, as promulgated by Lerner, was based on chickens in which there has been a high rate of inbreeding. In most human populations the level of inbreeding is far lower. There may be some exceptional populations such as, perhaps, these Indians. The average couple is related, as I said, at least as closely as first cousins once removed, which is a fair rate of inbreeding. One place to try to pursue this question would be in India. In some areas, uncle-niece marriage is 12%, as is first cousin marriage. That would be a nice place to work on the problem.

SECTION II

INFLUENCE OF NUTRITIONAL FACTORS DURING EARLY ADOLESCENCE ON REPRODUCTIVE EFFICIENCY

Isabelle Valadian
Robert B. Reed

From 1930 to 1956, Dr. Harold C. Stuart conducted his well known Longitudinal Studies of Child Health and Development in which he followed children from the prenatal to their 18th year period.[1] In 1965 these children had reached the age of 25 to 34 years, and we called them back to Boston for a follow-up entitled "Adult Health Related to Child Health and Development". The general objective of the follow-up was to determine the extent to which certain characteristics of the young adults could be predicted from the knowledge of their patterns of health and development during childhood.

As in the Longitudinal Studies, the follow-up is carried out by a team representing several disciplines: medicine, nutrition, dentistry, anthropology and social work.

One hundred and twenty-six of the 132 available subjects participated. They each spent two intensive days in Boston going through various examinations and interviews. This paper presents highlights of the investigation relating selected factors in childhood and adulthood to the reproductive ability of young women.

Sixty-four women participated in the follow-up. Fifty-nine had active sexual lives. Of these, 2 never conceived, 1 willfully ended her only pregnancy in the second month, so 56 shared a total of 209 pregnancies.

The reproductive histories were taken twice — once by the senior author and the other by the internist who performed the medical examination. In

Extensive financial support has been received from many sources to make possible the collection of the basic longitudinal data over the years since 1930. From July 1947 to June 1961 support was obtained from the Research Grant Division of the U.S. Public Health Service. The present support is from the National Institute of Child Health and Human Development — Grant HD 00772 –04.

addition, we tested the recall ability.

(1) The age of menarche asked by internist checked against childhood record. It shows no significant difference between mean age of menarche as recalled and observed. The correlation coefficient between menarcheal age in the childhood record and that recorded during the adult interview was +0.78.

(2) The same kind of result was obtained by checking the common childhood illnesses.

We characterized the reproductive quality according to events during prenatal course, labor, delivery and the outcome of each pregnancy.

The quantity and quality of prenatal care received was quite homogeneous. With one exception, all the women received early and regular care and all delivered in hospitals. Twenty-three women went uneventfully through all their pregnancies and gave birth to healthy babies, while 33 experienced difficulties of varying degree.

In order to facilitate analysis of reproduction and relate it to events of factors with which some relationship might rest, we developed a numerical rating of the reproductive experience for each woman. This led to a total score assessing a woman's entire reproductive experience on the basis of all her pregnancies and obtained a Reproductive Index. An index of 1 corresponds to normal, uneventful pregnancy, and the distribution of the indices was as follows: 40% with an index of 1; 20% between 1 and 1.75; and 40% over 1.75.

Example of a 1.8 Reproduction Index

Mrs. P. F. P. had 5 pregnancies; started prenatal care after missing first period; under the care of the same obstetrician (private).

Pregnancy I – Full term	Edema of legs after 7th month
	No toxemia, but on diet
	Forceps delivery – baby fine
Pregnancy II – Full term	Normal
Pregnancy III – Full term	Posterior presentation
Pregnancy IV – Miscarriage	3rd month
Pregnancy V – Full term	Normal

Example of a 3.3 Reproduction Index

Mrs. N. B. P. had 6 pregnancies; under the care of private obstetrician; started early.

Pregnancy I – Full term	A lot of vomiting during pregnancy
	Low forceps delivery

58

Pregnancy II – Miscarriage	3rd month
Pregnancy III – Full term	Normal
Pregnancy IV – Miscarriage	2nd month
Pregnancy V – Premature	1 month, weight 5 lbs., a couple of days in incubator
	Rough pregnancy, stained off and on
	Difficult pregnancy; subject qualified it as "brutal"
	Long labor, high temperature
	Postpartum kidney infection

We did not find significant association between reproduction and adult nutrition, smoking habits or food intake.

We did not find evidence of significant association between timing of menarche nor disturbances of menstruation through 18 years of age but we found a significant relationship between the quality of the first pregnancy and the length of time between menarche and conception. We found that 76% of the women who conceived for the first time within ten years after menarche went through that pregnancy with no problem. In contrast, 50% of the women who first conceived later than ten years experienced a normal pregnancy. This difference is significant. But the effect of this interval did not prove to be significant in the entire reproductive experience when subsequent pregnancies were considered.

We explored the influence of illness, nutrition and other factors that had occurred during the childhood of these women and we did find one interesting relationship. The protein intake during the entire 18 years was positively correlated with the outcome of pregnancies: 70% of women with high protein intake delivered all healthy babies (Table 1). Among women with low protein intake only 41% had all normal babies.

Because of the greater significance and implication of the protein intake, which we will see further, we would like to discuss the methodology of securing nutrition data.

We recognize dietery history, depending upon methods used, is subject to error. Therefore, great care was taken and a method developed which is known as the "Burke Dietary History Method." This method was developed in the early years of the Longitudinal Study to measure the average nutrient intake of an individual over a period of time, taking into account fluctuations in intake during the period covered by the history. The method includes the following steps:

TABLE 1

Relationship Between Protein Intake During Total Childhood
and Quality of Reproduction

Reproduction Index	Protein Intake (1 – 18 yrs.)		TOTAL
	Low	High	
1.0	9	12	21
> 1.0	20	11	31
TOTAL	29	23	52

$$X^2 = 2.381, \quad P > .05$$

mother (later the child and mother), and she recorded the pattern of eating both at and between meals in common household measures, and the extent to which the usual pattern of eating varied.

2. This interview was followed by a "cross check" designed to verify and classify the information obtained.

3. The nutritionist then calculated the amount of each food or food-group representative of the subject's average daily intake, using a standard set of procedures for translating lay descriptions of diets into scientific units of nutrient intake.

The reliability and validity of this dietary technique as a measuring device have been investigated and published.[3] It yields results which are satisfactorily reproducible.

The relationship of protein intake to reproductive performance was most striking when we focused upon the early adolescent period, from 8 to 12 years of age (Table 2). Eighty percent of women with a record of high protein intake (70 gm a day or more) during this early adolescent period had healthy babies in all pregnancies, whereas only 30% of women with low protein intake from 8 to 12 years had similarly successful reproductive performance.

The difference in protein intake history of women with good and bad reproductive performance appears in our data throughout the period from 2 to 12 years, although the statistical significance is most striking in the early adolescent period. After 12 years of age, there is no significant association with protein intake although the women with good reproductive performance still had slightly higher intakes (Table 3). Figures 1 – 6 illustrate individual protein intakes in the years before menarche for women who experienced various reproduction indices.

The protein intake findings were paralleled by associations with growth but not by relationships with development during childhood. Women with good and bad reproductive performance showed, on the average, practically identical ages at menarche and skeletal ages throughout childhood. However, women with good reproductive performance were approximately five centimeters taller than those with poor performance. This excess in height had been acquired almost entirely during the period from 2 to 12 years of age when these women had higher protein intakes. In fact, women with good reproductive performance showed slightly less growth from 12 to 18 years.

Review of Literature

Although there is fairly extensive literature on the effects of severe dietary restrictions during early development or during pregnancy, there are relatively few studies dealing with mild or moderate restriction and still fewer studies dealing with preadolescent or adolescent nutrition.

61

TABLE 2

Relationship Between Protein Intake at Early Adolescence
and Reproduction Index

Reproduction	Protein Intake (1 – 18 yrs.)		
Index	Low	High	TOTAL
1.0	7	15	22
> 1.75	17	4	21
TOTAL	24	19	43

$$X^2 = 10.518, \quad P < .05$$

TABLE 3

Relationship Between Protein Intake at Age 18 and Quality
of Reproduction

| Reproduction Index | Protein Intake (1 – 18 yrs.) | | TOTAL |
	Low	High	
1.0	10	11	21
1.0	18	13	31
	—	—	—
TOTAL	28	24	52

$$X^2 = 0.550, \quad P > .05$$

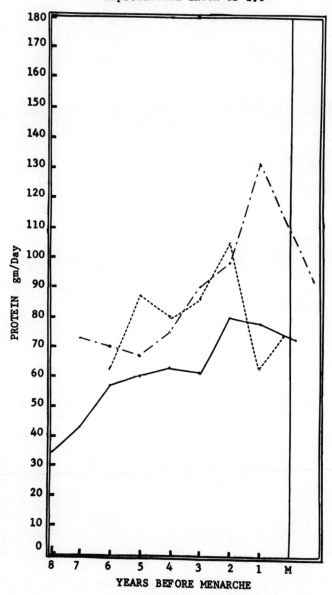

PROTEIN INTAKE BEFORE MENARCHE

Reproduction Index of 1.0

Figure 1

64

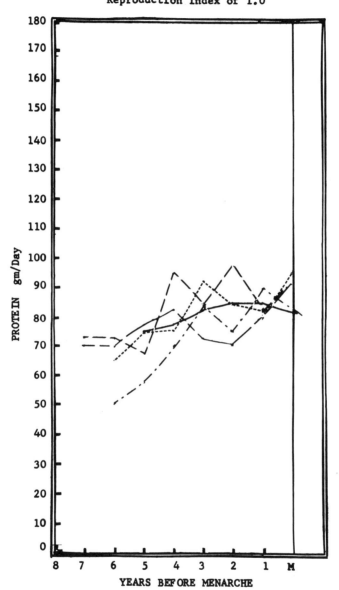

Figure 2

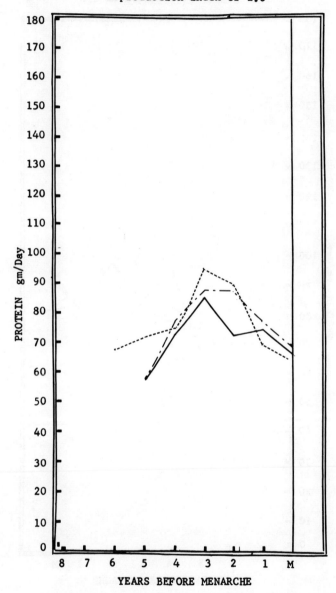

Figure 3

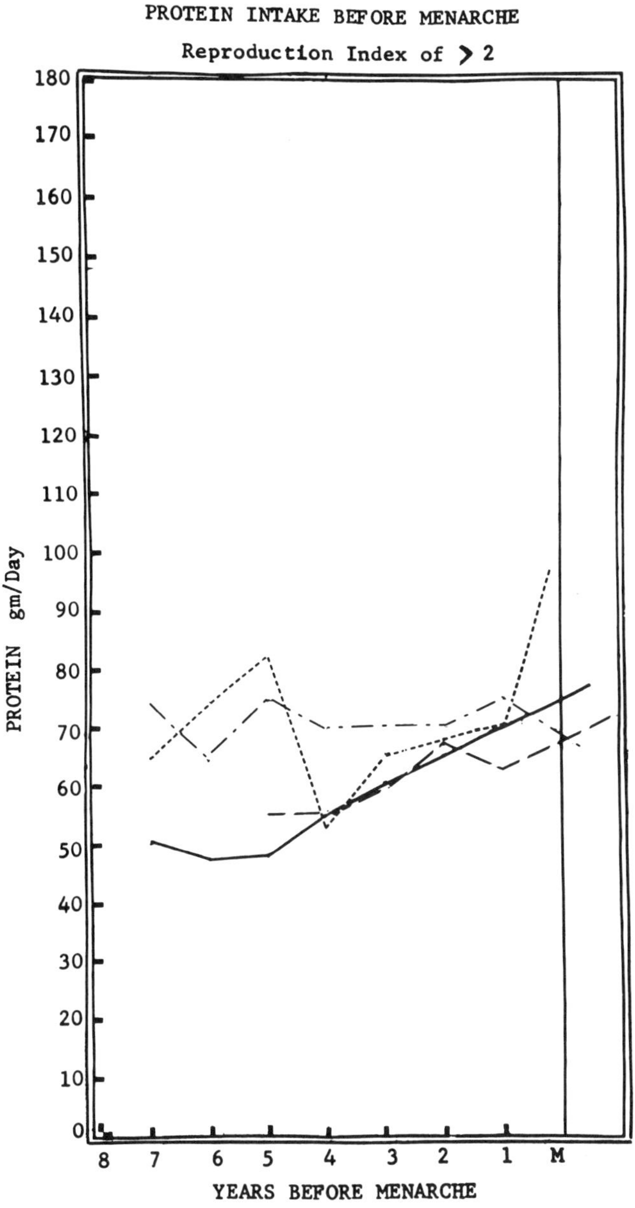

Figure 4

67

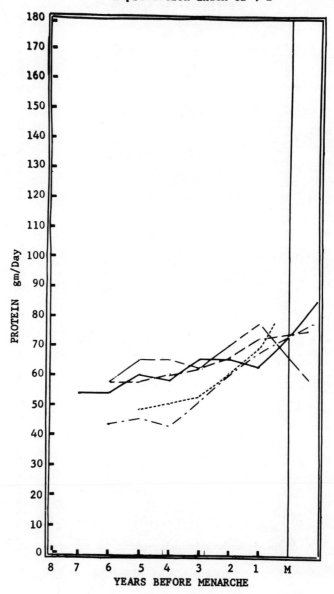

PROTEIN INTAKE BEFORE MENARCHE
Reproduction Index of > 2

YEARS BEFORE MENARCHE

Figure 5

68

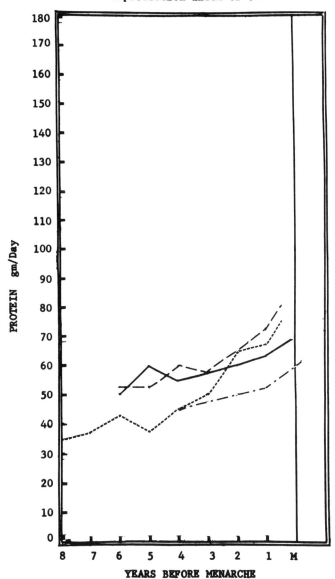

PROTEIN INTAKE BEFORE MENARCHE
Reproduction Index of > 3

YEARS BEFORE MENARCHE

PROTEIN gm/Day

Figure 6

69

The literature pertaining to livestock and laboratory animals has several studies.[4,5,6] In virtually all species studied (mostly lambs, pigs and rats), dietary deficiencies (calorie or protein) *occurring early in life:*

a. delay the onset of puberty;

b. decrease ovulation rate and

c. produce smaller youngs who have a higher preweaning death rate. The magnitude of these defects is dependent on the degree of deficiency.

In the human, we face a paucity of data. There are apparently no studies dealing with childhood or adolescent nutritional status on adult reproductive performance. Three studies report an association between these two: that is, childhood nutrition and adult reproduction and reached their conclusion in a rather speculative way.

Thompson[7] in Aberdeen says that the dietary intake during pregnancy can vary considerably in quantity and quality without adversely affecting the pregnancy outcome and that it is the previous nutritional status of the mother that is the determining factor.

Thompson[8] also found support for the importance of early nutritional status in the historical events in Britain in the past several decades: (1) Between 1940 – 1945 there was a rapid decrease in stillbirth rate which coincided with the improvement in the nutrition during pregnancy due to rationing allowances. However (2), following this there was little change despite an improvement in the levels of obstetric care. (3) In recent years there has again been a rapid decline. He speculates that this recent decline is due to the arrival of childbearing age of those who were better fed in World War II.

Another study by Aykroyd and Hossain[9] reports differences in infant death rates and especially neonatal for the Pakistan population in Bradford, Yorkshire, as compared with the Non-Asian rate. Stewart[10] suggests that this difference may reflect the poor nutritional status of the mothers during their childhood and adolescence in Pakistan.

Summary and Conclusion

While the basic finding of association between childhood nutrition and reproduction is statistically significant in our data, the problem is sufficiently complex to require considerably more study before the relationship can be said to be firmly established or clearly understood. We are inclined to see that nutritional variations even within "normal" limits prior to menarche may play an important part in establishing the capacity of a girl to reproduce satisfactorily in later life. We believe that our data suggest, although they certainly do not prove, that this effect is most prominent during the 4 to 5 years immediately prior to menarche, and that it is related to aspects of the development of the reproductive system over and above the phenomenon of growth in size and in influence on the functioning of their organs.

REFERENCES

1. H.C. Stuart *et al.*, *Monograph of Soc. for Res. in Child Devel. 4*, serial 20, No. 1, Monograph I, 1939.

2. A. Damon, S.T. Damon, R.B. Reed and I. Valadian, *Hum. Biol. 41*, 161, 1969.

3. R.B. Reed and B.S. Burke, *Am. J. Pub. Health 44*, 1015, 1954.

4. R.J.C. Stewart and H.G. Sheppard, *Brit. J. Nutr. 25*, 175, 1971.

5. S.R. Gupta and B. Lacy, *Indian J. Med. Res. 55*, 904, 1967.

6. S.R. Gupta and B. Christie, *Indian J. Med. Res. 56*, 114, 1968.

7. A.M. Thomson, *Brit. J. Nutr. 12*, 446, 1958; *Brit. J. Nutr. 13*, 190 - 204, 509 - 525, 1959.

8. A.M. Thomson and F.E. Hytten, *Proc. 7th Int. Cong. Nutr.*, Hamburg, 1966, New York, Pergamon Press, p. 67, 1967.

9. W.R. Aykroyd and M.A. Hossain, *Brit. Med. J. 1*, 42, 1967.

10. R.J.C. Stewart, *Proc. R. Soc. Med. 61*, 1292, 1968.

MATERNAL FACTORS IN C.N.S. MALFORMATIONS: THE COHORT APPROACH

Dwight T. Janerich

Introduction

Attempts to resolve the issue of genetic versus environmental explanations for most of the common major congenital malformations in man has produced considerable, but fruitless, debate. Polygenic thresholds with environmental interaction has evolved as a compromising middle ground. This mechanism is flexible enough to fit almost any observed pattern of family aggregation of congenital disease, but is quite unhelpful in suggesting environmental factors which can be manipulated to provide some measure of prevention or control.

The consensus opinion suggests a combined genetic and environmental etiology. In the forseeable future, it seems more reasonable to attempt to control the occurrence of these defects through identification and manipulation of relevant environmental factors, rather than to depend on the relatively uncertain possibilities of active or passive genetic manipulation. This presentation will be directed toward the use of epidemiologic methods to expand our knowledge of the way in which environmental factors cause major congenital malformations in human populations. We recognize two ways in which environmental factors can affect the occurrence of congenital malformations. Evidence from both human and animal studies has shown how environmental agents can act during pregnancy to cause congenital defects. In addition, animal studies have shown that environmental factors can affect the female during early life and produce a pronounced effect on teratogenic susceptibility during the reproductive period. In epidemiologic terms this is referred to as a generation effect. This implies that the effect in question can be attributed to early exposure to environmental conditions whose influence persists through life, in this case, the reproductive life.

Background on Anencephaly and Spina Bifida

Among the major congenital malformations which affect man, the central nervous system malformations are the most easily diagnosed and most

73

efficiently recorded at the time of birth. They are an appropriate focus for an examination of the issue of genetic versus environmental factors in the etiology of congenital defects in man. Two of these malformations – anencephaly and spina bifida – appear to be etiologically similar. This conclusion is partly based on the similarity of their epidemiologic patterns. On a world-wide basis, they are among the most common and most severe congenital malformations to affect man.

The literature contains a number of hypotheses relating to the etiology of these malformations, but definitive evidence supporting any one of them is lacking. In general, these hypotheses can be classified as either genetic or environmental in nature. Each category of epidemiologic evidence tends to support either the genetic or environmental side of the argument. Unfortunately, the weight of the epidemiologic evidence is split between support for the genetic and support for the environmental side of the controversy.

Following is a list of the six major epidemiologic characteristics which are associated with the occurrence of anencephaly and spina bifida.

Family Recurrence – After the occurrence of an index case in a family, the risk of having another child affected by anencephaly or spina bifida is five percent, substantially higher than the risk in the general population. Carter has shown the recurrence risk to be slightly higher after the occurrence of a second affected case in a family.[1] Falconer has developed a mathematical model which explains this level of recurrence risk on the basis of a polygenic mode of inheritance.[2] It has been concluded that the family recurrence patterns observed for anencephaly and spina bifida suggest a genetic etiology. However, the development of a model based on empirical evidence, which has the capability of quantitatively predicting the recurrence risk of a particular event should not be considered as synonymous with an understanding of the underlying biological mechanism which produces that event. MacMahon and Yen have noted that the recurrence of environmental factors within the family setting could also explain the observed familial pattern.[15] In addition, Nance has observed that the familial patterns are also consistent with cytoplasmic inheritance.[3]

Twin Concordance – Although there is some controversy on the issue, the concordance rate for anencephaly and spina bifida appears to be higher among monozygotic twins than among dizygotic twins. Since monozygotic twins are identical from a genetic point of view, while dizygotic twins are not, the available evidence seems to suggest a genetic etiology. However, the fact that the majority of affected monozygotic twin pairs are not concordant for anencephaly or spina bifida suggests that the genetic factors play less than a predominant role in the etiology of these malformations.

Ethnic Effect – The observation that the prevalence of these malformations

74

among births, varies greatly between various population groups, suggests a genetic role in the etiology of anencephaly and spina bifida. These differences are often quite large. For example, in parts of Great Britain the prevalence of these malformations is five times as great as that found in Israel.

Socio-economic Effect — Repeated studies have shown an inverse relationship between the prevalence of these malformations and the parents' socio-economic status. Since socio-economic factors govern the standard of living, and therefore the family's environment, the relationship is taken to suggest an environmental etiology. Lowe has noted that in South Wales — some part of the poverty complex is clearly involved in the etiology of neural tube defects because the prevalence seems to be becoming less as the standard of living rises.[4]

Birth Order and Maternal Age Effect — The risk of having a child with anencephaly or spina bifida varies with mothers' age and number of previous births. Since the genes of each parent are equally dispersed among their children at conception, this association is taken to suggest an environmental etiology. However, McKeown and Record have noted that these associations are of little interest unless their significance is further explored.[5]

Epidemic Waves — One of the most curious and striking epidemiologic features of anencephaly and spina bifida, is the tendency of these malformations to appear in epidemic patterns. Two types of these epidemics have been identified, (a) small, local, short-term epidemics and (b) large epidemic waves which span decades. A number of these small epidemics have been investigated and reported in the literature.[6] We are presently investigating two such small epidemics which occurred in New York State during the last four years. Unfortunately, none of these investigations seem to definitely pinpoint a specific, causal, environmental agent.

The second type, or large epidemic wave, has only recently been recognized. MacMahon and Yen have described a mammoth epidemic which spanned approximately thirty years, from 1920 to 1950.[7] The available data is limited, but suggests that the epidemic occurred at least in the Northeastern United States and may also have occurred in other parts of the world.[8] Several environmental explanations have been hypothesized but the precise cause of the epidemic remains unknown.

Therefore, among the six major epidemiologic characteristics which we have discussed, three suggest an environmental etiology and three suggest a genetic etiology. From the available evidence it is not possible to decide between these two alternatives.

In the remaining portion of this presentation we will examine the available data on the secular trends, or epidemics, of these defects. In addition, we will examine the relationship between maternal age and the risk of these malformations. Our purpose will be to produce evidence to help identify possible causal environmental agents. In particular, we will try to show that it is reasonable to consider the possibility that the environmental factors which produce these malformations have their origins early in the mother's life.

Epidemics

Figure 1 illustrates data from Boston Lying-In Hospital and Providence Lying-In Hospital from the turn of the century through 1965. The data is from a report by MacMahon and Yen and describes the epidemic which peaked in the early 1930's.[7] The prevalence rates are for anencephaly and spina bifida combined, and are presented in five-year intervals. The authors suggested that the peak of the epidemic occurred in the early 1930's with the duration being from 1920 to 1949. In addition to the distinct peak in the rates in the early 1930's, two other features of the data stand out. First, the rate in Boston Lying-In is consistently lower than in Providence Lying-In, during both epidemic and non-epidemic periods. Second, there is a distinct secondary peak in the Providence data in the early 1940's which is not noticeable in the Boston data. We will refer to this secondary peak in the Providence data again later using data from Boston which was presented by Naggan.

Data presented by Rodgers and Morris[8] describing infant mortality in England and Wales from 1850 to 1960 suggests that a somewhat similar epidemic occurred in those countries about the same time. This suggests that the epidemic may not have been limited to the Northeastern United States.

The data illustrated in Figure 2 was taken from a report by Naggan, and describes the prevalence of anencephaly and spina bifida among births in four large Boston hospitals between 1930 and 1965.[9] Naggan's report predates the report by MacMahon and Yen which recognized that the declining rate from 1930 to 1949 represented the waning of an epidemic. The illustration clearly shows the uninterrupted decline from 1930 to 1949 which was later to become recognized as the decline of the epidemic. We can note that there is no distinct secondary peak in the early 1940's. Figure 3 shows the same data subdivided by father's occupational class according to Warner's procedure for measurement of social class. The lowest occupational classes – designated as O. C. 6 and 7 – are on the upper grid with progressively higher occupational classes on each lower grid. An examination of this illustration shows that the peak in the early 1930's is seen in all occupational classes, while the lowest occupational class also has a distinct peak in the early 1940's similar to that which was seen in the Providence data described by MacMahon and Yen.[7]

This suggests that the 1930 peak was caused by some phenomenon which

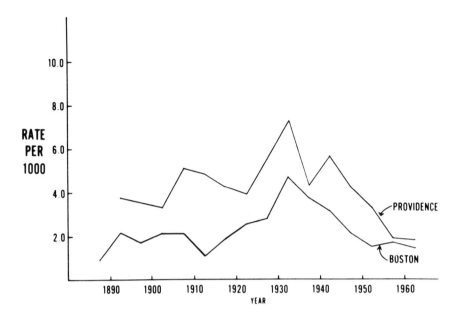

Fig. 1. Rate of anencephaly and spina bifida, 1890 to 1965, in Boston Lying-in and Providence Lying-in, from data of MacMahon and Yen.[7]

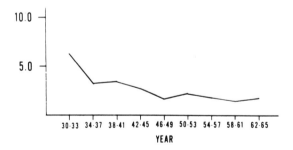

Fig. 2. Rate of anencephaly and spina bifida, 1930 to 1965, in four Boston hospitals, from data of Naggan.[9]

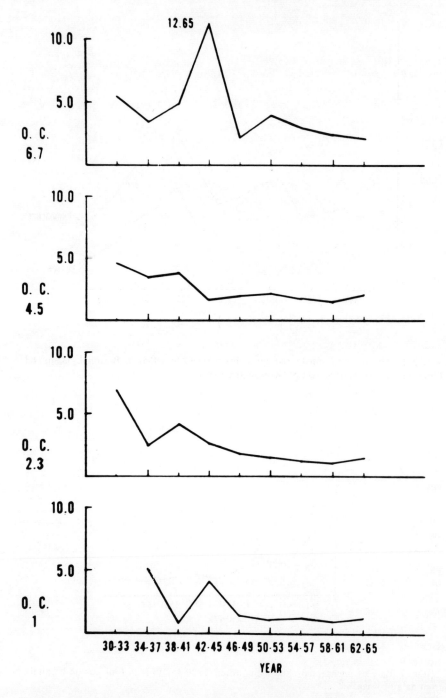

Fig. 3. Rate of anencephaly and spina bifida, 1930 to 1965, in four Boston hospitals, by parental occupational class, from data of Naggan.[9]

affected all social classes while the secondary peak in the early 1940's was the result of some phenomenon which was most severely experienced by the lower socio-economic classes but not limited to the lower socio-economic classes. The fact that the overall prevalence of these malformations was higher in the Providence Lying-In data as compared to Boston Lying-In data suggested that the patients in the former hospital generally came from a lower social class. MacMahon and Yen, in reporting the epidemic, suggested that socio-economic differences may be responsible for the difference in prevalence between the two hospitals. Since Naggan's data from Boston shows the peak in the early 1940's was limited to the lower socio-economic groups, the fact that the peak in the early 1940's appears in the overall Providence data seems to confirm that the data from Providence is from a generally lower socio-economic segment of the population.

Maternal Age in Anencephaly and Spina Bifida

Before continuing our examination of the available data on the epidemic, we would like to digress temporarily to develop a line of reasoning which will bear on our interpretation of the data from the epidemic. To do this, we will examine the relationship between maternal age and risk of delivering a child with anencephaly or spina bifida. There is considerable variability, between studies, in the reported pattern of this relationship.

Fedrick has reviewed the literature on the relationship between maternal age and anencephaly.[10] In a number of studies the risk was seen to increase as maternal age increased. Some other studies showed the risk to decrease as maternal age increased. However, the majority of studies showed the risk to follow a "U" shaped pattern — that is, a high risk in younger and older mothers, with the lowest risk occurring in the middle reproductive years, specifically 25–29 years of age.

We believe there is a discernible overall pattern to this apparent inconsistency, and we believe that an understanding of that pattern could provide us with a valuable clue to the etiology of these malformations.

An interesting contrast emerges as one examines the reported maternal age effect in areas where the incidence is high, compared to areas where the incidence is low. South Wales and Israel are examples of these extremes. Table 1 describes the rate of anencephaly and spina bifida in South Wales from 1956–1962.[1] The rate of both malformations during that period was 7.7 malformed infants per thousand births. During the period 1958–1968 in Israel the rate was 1.5 malformed infants per 1000 births.[11] The rate in South Wales was five times as great as that found in Israel. Figure 4 shows a ratio of observed to expected frequencies of these malformations within the standard maternal age grouping for the data from South Wales. The typical

TABLE 1

Prevalence of Anencephaly and Spina Bifida per 1000 Births

Malformations	South Wales Carter *et al.* 1956–1962	Israel Naggan 1958–1968
Anencephaly	3.54	0.86
Spina Bifida	4.13	0.60
Both	7.67	1.46

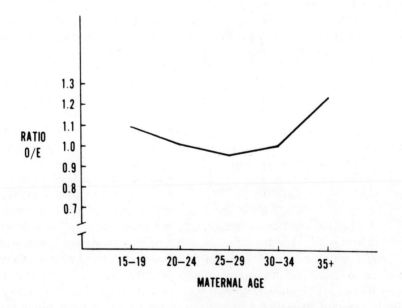

Fig. 4. Ratio of observed to expected for anencephaly and spina bifida in South Wales, 1956-62, by maternal age, from data of Carter, David and Laurence.[1]

80

"U" shaped pattern can be seen. (The format in which the data was presented in this report required the use of the ratios rather than rates. Although ratios tend to minimize the strength of the relationship, they do not distort the pattern of the relationship.) There is a steady decline in the risk from 15 to 19 years of age, and in the older age groups there is a progressive increase in the risk.

Figure 5 shows the maternal age-specific risk from Naggan's data from Israel.[11] The age intervals are the same except that the under-25-year age groups were consolidated into a single group. The declining risk through 29 years of age seen in the South Wales data is not in evidence in the data from Israel. However, the higher risk among older mothers is present in both data sets.

The "U" shaped pattern which was seen in South Wales and which is most frequently observed in other areas, is not suggestive of any obvious single, biological phenomenon. A separate high risk among older mothers and younger mothers suggests either that multiple phenomenon are operating in the causation of these malformations or that this type of analysis in some way produces an artificial bimodality. If we accept the data sets from South Wales and Israel as valid estimates of the maternal age effect in these two countries, it becomes reasonable to ask why they vary. One of the most evident differences is that, in South Wales, where the overall rate of these malformations ranks among the highest of any place in the world, there is a declining risk from the youngest to 30-year-old mothers. In Israel, where the overall rate ranks among the lowest of any place in the world, there is no evidence of this decline.

In reflecting on this difference, it seems reasonable to ask whether the observed difference is the result of some change in an etiologic factor which is peculiar to that population, or is it a function of the relative overall frequency of these malformations? To attempt to answer this question, we decided to examine the maternal age effect in data on spina bifida from New York State. Birth record data on anencephaly and spina bifida has been available since 1945. During that period the rate of neural tube closure defects declined dramatically from 1945 to 1949 and reached somewhat of a plateau in more recent years. As was mentioned earlier, the dramatic decline has now been established by MacMahon and Yen to be the tail end of an epidemic of these malformations.[7]

Figure 6 shows the declining rate seen in upstate New York compared with data from Boston Lying-In Hospital and Providence Lying-In Hospital.[7] The rate in the Providence data is consistently higher than that found in either Boston or upstate New York. The pattern of the decline in each case is quite similar in that the decline was greater in the earlier part of the period than in

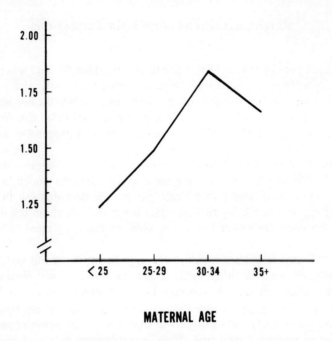

Fig. 5. Rate of anencephaly and spina bifida, 1945 to 1968, in Israel, from data of Naggan.[11]

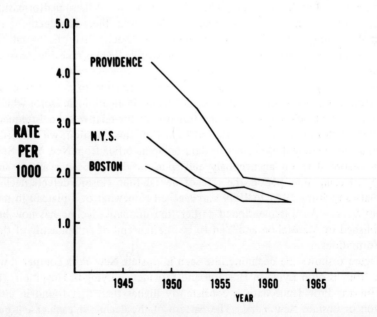

Fig. 6. Rate of anencephaly and spina bifida, 1945 to 1965, in Boston and Providence, from MacMahon and Yen[7] and upstate New York birth records.

82

the later part of the period.

In the following discussion we will examine the maternal age effect which was reported for spina bifida. Anencephaly is excluded because it has been independently studied by us and reported elsewhere.[12] All diagnostic categories generally listed under the heading of spina bifida are included.

Figure 7 shows the maternal age-specific rate of spina bifida for five-year intervals from 1945 to 1964. The distinct "U" shaped pattern which was seen in the 1945–49 period became less distinct but was still discernible in each succeeding five-year interval. Figure 8 shows the maternal age effect from 1965–70. The "U" shaped pattern has essentially disappeared. Although the risk is generally higher among the older age groups, there is no sign of a consistent decline from 15 to 29 years of age as we saw in our earlier data, as well as in the data from South Wales.

As the overall prevalence in New York declined, the high risk among younger mothers diminished and the maternal age pattern began to resemble that which was seen in the Israeli data. This type of change suggests that the relationship between maternal age and risk of these malformations is a function of the overall prevalence of these malformations rather than the specific population in which it occurs. This conclusion does not seem unreasonable if one is considering an environmental rather than a genetic etiology.

This change in the maternal age effect could be produced by some change in the basic underlying etiologic mechanism. However, it could also be an artifact produced by a known methodological deficiency in the procedure by which we traditionally determine the relationship between maternal age and the risk of delivering a defective child.

Frequently, limited resources and limited data have forced us to take a shortcut in determining the risk of defective offspring in relation to maternal age. Ideally, we should follow a group of women through their reproductive careers, either prospectively or retrospectively, and determine the risk of delivering a defective offspring at sequential age intervals. This method is time consuming and expensive and therefore avoided. Instead, we substitute cross-sectional data, that is, data which is produced in a short-time interval from various groups of women at various stages of their reproductive lives. We take one group of women who are 15–19 years of age at a specific time and determine their risk of delivering a malformed child. We then take a different group which is 20–24 years of age during that same specific time period and measure their risk. We repeat this procedure subsequentially through the reproductive years. We then assemble the individual risks from each age-specific group and label the results as the maternal age-specific risk of delivering a child with that particular defect. If we can be sure that the maternal age-specific risk does not change over time, this is a perfectly

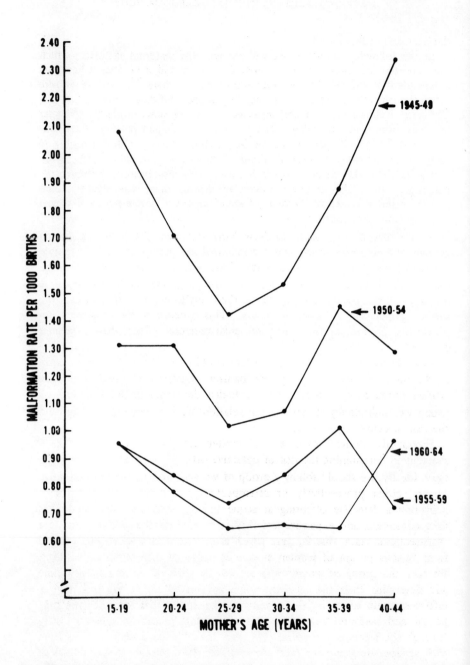

Fig. 7. Rate of spina bifida, 1945 to 1964, by maternal age, from upstate New York birth records.

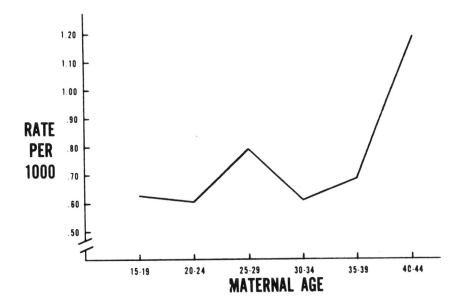

Fig. 8. Rate of spina bifida, 1965 to 1970, by maternal age, from upstate New York birth records.

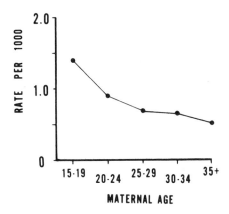

Fig. 9. Cohort specific rate of spina bifida, by maternal age, for mothers born from 1931 to 1935.[14]

adequate procedure. However, if that risk does change over time, the results of substituting cross-sectional for longitudinal studies can be quite misleading. The problems created by this type of methodological shortcut have been recognized in studies of physical growth data.[13] In periods during which the age-specific growth rate had changed, the results of cross-sectional and longitudinal studies have been shown to differ. A similar but probably more serious situation could occur in data such as we are discussing.

We have seen that the cross-sectional view of data describing the relationship seems to be a function of the overall prevalence of these malformations. Under these circumstances it does not seem unreasonable to suspect that the substitution of cross-sectional for longitudinal data has produced unreliable results.

Using data which was available in New York State, we have attempted to do longitudinal studies of the relationship between maternal age and risk of having a child with anencephaly or spina bifida.[12,14] We assembled data for individual, birth-year related cohorts of women — for the portion of their reproductive lives which occurred between 1945 and 1970. Nineteen forty-five marks the first year for which malformation information was available on birth records. Analyzing data from the longitudinal aspect produced a substantially different result than was obtained by the cross-sectional approach which was described above. Figure 9 is an example of that analysis for spina bifida alone.[14] It illustrates the cohort-specific risk of delivering a child with spina bifida for those women who were born from 1931 to 1935. The "U" shaped pattern which was seen in the cross-sectional approach discussed earlier, was not seen in the longitudinal approach. The longitudinal studies suggested that the risk declined with increasing maternal age, and that the "U" shaped, cross-sectional pattern produced by the cross-sectional studies was the result of higher cohort-specific risks among women born earlier in time.

This observation is indeed puzzling. In theory, the method which was used in this study is logically more sound than that which is used in the traditional cross-sectional approach. The expected degree of preciseness of data assembled in this way has not yet been established, but a lack of precision is not likely to produce such a consistent artifact. Before a conclusion can be reached on the apparent ambiguity between the longitudinal and cross-sectional we will have to better understand how the secular trend and the cohort-specific risk interact. The latter is a difficult task since we do not yet know what factors determine the secular trend.

To our knowledge there are only two published reports which offer data that can be used to examine the validity of our observation. These studies refer to time factors within families. Although the data in these studies was assembled in the same type of format as we have used, it is similar enough for us to use the data to comment on the relationship between maternal age and risk of having a child with anencephaly or spina bifida. Furthermore, the data is limited to high-risk families, thus avoiding the possible confounding factors inherent in general population studies.

In the first study, Yen and MacMahon showed a slight decline in the family recurrence risk with time since the birth of an index case.[15] This decline is directly compatible with a decreasing risk as maternal age increased. In that study, the authors assumed that the decline was a function of the declining secular trend which occurred through a segment of the time period under study. However, they did not pursue evidence to support that assumption. In the second study, Carter, David and Laurence[1] presented data from a family study in South Wales. They selected their index cases from births occurring from 1956 to 1962. They examined the recurrence risks in these families. Among their results they note that the cumulative risk to sibs born before their index case was slightly higher compared with the risk to sibs born after the index case. This data also suggests that the risk of having a child with anencephaly and spina bifida is higher at younger maternal ages than at older maternal ages. Their data was not affected by a declining secular risk in the same way as the data of Yen and MacMahon. The early part of the period from which they selected their index cases was the peak of an epidemic. The data in these two studies cannot be used to imply definitive proof of a decreasing risk with increasing maternal age, but they do provide some supporting evidence for our contention. At this point, we should mention that the repeated observation of an increased risk of anencephaly and spina bifida among first births is directly compatible with a risk pattern which decreases with increasing maternal age.

Aside from the need to seek further corroboration of these findings we are faced with the need to explain the question – why does the cross-sectional analysis show a "U" shaped risk pattern? We believe the explanation is that each cohort has a specific, relative risk which is related to the woman's year of birth. To show this we can examine the age-specific risk in the 35-plus age category of each cohort for which we have data.

As we can see from Table 2, each succeeding elder cohort has a progressively higher age-specific risk. If the risk of each individual mother is a composite function of her age at the time of birth of her child and her cohort-specific risk – then a situation in which the cohort-specific risk was, or had recently been, declining would artificially produce a "U" shaped risk pattern in the cross-sectional format. This could occur even though the actual risk declined with increasing maternal age.

If, in the final determination, the risk of anencephaly and spina bifida is

TABLE 2

Rate of Spina Bifida by Mother's Year of Birth for 35+ Years of Age

Mother's Year of Birth	Rate per 1000 Births
1901 – 1910	1.96
1911 – 1915	1.61
1916 – 1920	1.21
1921 – 1925	.90
1926 – 1930	.81

shown to decline with increasing maternal age, it will be reasonable to conclude that we are dealing with a generation effect.

Our observation, if it is supported by further study, must have an interpretation before it can prove to be biologically or epidemiologically meaningful. We suggest that the cohort-specific risk is related to the mother's year of birth because it reflects the effect of the environmental factors which were prevalent during the early part of the mother's life. These factors, although not yet identifiable, must have a lasting effect on her risk of delivering a child with anencephaly or spina bifida. The biological mechanism might be similar to the environmentally-induced cytoplasmic or maternal effect which was demonstrated by Verrusio, Pollard and Fraser.[16] This mechanism seems to provide a reasonable model for anencephaly and spina bifida since Nance[3] has shown that a cytoplasmic or maternal factor may be responsible for the familial occurrence pattern.

In support of our contention, we would like to note a conclusion reached by Anderson, Baird and Thomson[17] from a small study reported in 1958. They found an unusually large number of short women among mothers who had offspring affected with neural tube closure defects. They concluded,

> "... within *the lower social classes,* it is these under-
> sized women, stunted by the environment in which
> they have grown, who have the highest incidences
> of stillbirth and infant death due to malformation of
> the central nervous system."

Perhaps the environmental factors affecting high risk mothers early in their lives are serious enough to interfere with their own normal growth, or the growth retardation causes alteration which predisposes the woman to the factors which cause these malformations.

Each of the two types of analysis which we have employed here have yielded at least one suggestion as to the nature of possible environmental agents which might be causally involved in the etiology of anencephaly and spina bifida. The serial cross-sectional analysis produced results which suggests that a high prevalence, or epidemic, of these malformations is due to some factor which has a greater effect on younger mothers than on older mothers. The longitudinal analysis produced results which suggest that the environmental factors operate early in the mother's life. Armed with these suggestions we will attempt to further explore the available data relative to the epidemics of anencephaly and spina bifida which occurred during the early part of this century.

Maternal Age Effect and Epidemic

MacMahon and Yen suggested that the extent of the epidemic or epidemics was probably from 1920–1949.[7] An examination of this data suggests that the extent of the epidemic may be somewhat questionable but there can be little doubt that the major peak occurred about 1930. MacMahon and Yen indicated that the series of high rates which formed the peak of the epidemic occurred in 1929 to 1932. The data presented by Naggan suggest that the secondary peak which occurred in the early to middle 1940's occurred primarily in the lower occupational or socio-economic class.

In a search to identify events which may have influenced the prevalence of relevant environmental factors, we can find at least four major historical events which occurred in the first half of the century and which could be related to these epidemics. World War I and World War II certainly qualify as major historical events which had significant effects on human environment. The American involvement in World War I began in 1917 and ended in 1918. The American involvement in World War II started in 1941 and ended in 1945. The third event which occurred during this time was the influenza pandemic of 1918. It was one of the most significant epidemics of infectious disease ever recorded and was accompanied, over the course of several years, by a series of significant epidemic peaks in mortality from influenza. This was an obviously more severe form of influenza than we have experienced in more recent times. The fourth major event which occurred in the first half of the century was the great Depression which started just after the stock market crash in 1929 and reached its worst stages in 1933–34 when unemployment reached its highest levels. We will first examine these events in relation to their possible direct influence on the affected pregnancies which produced the epidemic.

World War I does not appear to coincide in time with any portion of the epidemic. However, prohibition of alcohol started during World War I and continued afterward by constitutional amendment until repeal of that amendment in 1933. MacMahon and Yen suggested that some contaminant of illicit alcohol may have been responsible for the early part of the epidemic. This suggestion seems reasonable. This hypothesis may be consistent with our observation that the responsible environmental factor had a greater effect among younger mothers than among older mothers. However, the authors noted that the peak of the epidemic occurred before the repeal of prohibition. It is also difficult to explain a secondary peak and the extent of the epidemic through 1949 by this mechanism. Furthermore, this mechanism would not be helpful in explaining the epidemic which apparently occurred in England and South Wales at a similar period of time.

The lower socio-economic groups are known to have a high prevalence of anencephaly and spina bifida among their offspring. It has been suggested that the epidemic might be explained by factors related to the deterioration of the socio-economic conditions associated with the great Depression. This illustration of the data shows a somewhat close correspondence in time between the peak of the epidemic and the worst part of the Depression. However, the correspondence in time does not seem to be close enough. The major peak in the epidemic occurred from 1929—1932, but the worst part of the Depression — as measured by unemployment — did not occur until 1933 and 1934. Again, the duration does not fit. The epidemic started in the early 1920's — too early to be explained by any effect from the Depression. For one event to cause another, the causal event must occur at the time of, or before, the event which is hypothesized to result from it.

The mid-point of World War II seems to correspond with the mid-point of the secondary peak of the epidemic. It seems possible that some environmental disturbance, perhaps some nutritional deficiency associated with World War II, could explain the secondary peak. It also seems possible that this disturbance could have affected the lower socio-economic classes most severely but this type of disturbance probably would have disappeared well before 1949. In searching for additional hypothetical factors we should consider one which would affect younger mothers more than older mothers.

In suggesting possible causes, we have not yet considered the possibility of a generation effect caused by an environmental exposure early in life. An event which produced a lasting effect by acting on a female at about the time of puberty would exert its maximum effect on the birth population approximately twelve years later. It would also begin to exert its influence on the birth population soon after its occurrence. It would have its final effect on the birth population some thirty years after the event, as the affected cohort reached the end of its reproductive life. The magnitude of the effect throughout the epidemic would be governed to some degree by the relationship between maternal age and the risk of a defective offspring.

The first peak in the epidemic of anencephaly and spina bifida occurred eleven years after the great influenza pandemic. Both the influenza pandemic and the malformation epidemic affected all socio-economic groups. Therefore, in terms of time and population affected, the relationship between the influenza pandemic and the primary peak in the malformation epidemic are consistent with a cohort mechanism.

The secondary peak in the malformation epidemic occurred about ten or eleven years after the worst part of the great Depression. The secondary peak was most severely felt among the lower socio-economic groups. If we assume that the effects of the Depression were most severely felt among the lower socio-economic groups, then in terms of time and population affected, the relationship between the worst period of the Depression and the secondary peak in the malformations epidemic are also consistent with a cohort mechanism. Our evidence can only suggest that an association exists. The nature of the association is not apparent. Further study is needed. To decipher the meaning of the conflicting data on the effect of maternal age on the risk of delivering a child with anencephaly or spina bifida is a key step in resolving the epidemiologic aspects of the issue. If the risk declines with increasing maternal age, then we are probably dealing with a generation effect. If the pattern of risk is "U" shaped, then the environmental component of the etiologic mechanism is probably some factor or agent which affects younger mothers more than older mothers. To resolve this issue we must provide a definitive determination of the relationship between maternal age and risk of delivering a child with a neural tube closure defect.

In summary, we have tried to use a study of the effect of maternal age on the risk of delivering a child with anencephaly and spina bifida to provide clues to the nature of the environmental factors which operate in the etiology of anencephaly and spina bifida. We believe that the situation suggests some type of generation effect. Perhaps, in man as in laboratory animals, the susceptibility to teratogens can itself be environmentally determined.[16]

REFERENCES

1. C.O. Carter, P.A. David and K.M. Laurence, *J. Med. Genet. 5,* 81, 1968.

2. D.S. Falconer, *Ann. Hum. Genet. 29,* 51, 1965.

3. W.E. Nance, *Nature 224,* 373, 1965.

4. C.R. Lowe, *Brit. Med. J. 3,* 515, 1972.

5. T. McKeown and R.G. Record, *Am. J. Hum. Genet. 8,* 8, 1956.

6. J. Siemiatycki and A.D. McDonald, *Brit. J. Prev. Soc. Med. 26,* 19, 1972.

7. B. MacMahon and S. Yen, *Lancet 1,* 31, 1971.

8. S.C. Rogers and M. Moris, *Ann. Hum. Genet., Lond. 34,* 295, 1971.

9. L. Naggan, *Am. J. Epidemiol. 89,*154, 1969.

10. J. Fedrick, *Ann. Hum. Genet., Lond. 34,* 31, 1970.

11. L. Naggan, *Pediat. 47,* 577, 1971.

12. D.T. Janerich, *Am. J. Epidemiol. 95,* 319, 1972.

13. J.M. Tanner, *Hum. Biol. 23,* 93, 1951.

14. D.T. Janerich, *Am. J. Epidemiol. 96,* 389, 1972.

15. S. Yen and B. MacMahon, *Lancet 11,* 623, 1968.

16. A.C. Verrusio, D.R. Pollard and F.C. Fraser, *Science 160,* 206, 1968.

17. W.J.R. Anderson, D. Baird and A.M. Thomson, *Lancet 1,* 1304, 1958.

RECORD LINKAGE – ITS ROLE IN CONGENITAL DEFECT RESEARCH

Howard B. Newcombe

INTRODUCTION

Investigations of congenital defects in man frequently require that a great deal of time be spent in searching for facts about individual people which are known to have been recorded somewhere but are not quickly accessible to the investigator. As a result, many of the important questions remain unanswered, not because the information doesn't exist, but simply because it is fragmented, widely scattered and deeply buried in various massive accumulations of records. The kinds of information I have in mind relate mainly to the successions of events in the lives of individual people which, if brought together in the form of follow-up histories, could provide clues concerning cause-and-effect relationships.

I am going to ask you to consider what advantages might accrue from a deliberate attempt to ensure in the future that the relevant records, many of which are already being manipulated and stored by computers, become organized to permit rapid access and to facilitate the systematic extraction of individual follow-up histories throughout whole populations.

The essential feature of such an operation has been termed "record linkage". By this is meant the bringing together of two or more independently recorded facts about the same individual or family. The techniques for integrating the diverse files in which the source records occur, and for matching and linking together those records which relate to the same individuals or families, have now been developed to a high level of sophistication. As a result, the chief remaining impediments to record linkage are organizational rather than technological.

For the purposes of this symposium, it may be appropriate to consider first what kinds of relevant information could be made available through this approach. Many of the questions that come to mind are fairly obvious, and what will also be obvious is that the answers currently available are far from satisfactory.

I am thinking of such questions as:

a. How many cases of birth defects are there?
b. What are the causes of the defects?
c. How seriously do they affect the lives of the people concerned?
d. How effective are the available methods of treatment and management?
e. And, what are the social costs of failures to prevent the defects and treat them at the appropriate times?

These questions will be considered in greater detail in relation to the data obtainable from particular kinds of health records, when arranged to permit the extraction of individual histories of health events throughout whole populations.

CASE FINDINGS

There are numerous estimates, for example, of the individual and combined frequencies of congenital defects in birth populations. No single source of information, however, is adequate by itself as a basis for such estimates. This is true of virtually all *ad hoc* surveys of newborn infants, of routine physicians' notifications of births on which there is a question concerning birth anomalies, of hospital records, and of registrations of deaths on which congenital malformations are mentioned as a cause. Only a fraction of the birth defects are actually lethal, and many of those which involve internal organs, or affect learning ability, may not be discovered until some time after birth. Taken together, however, the various sources tend to complement one another.

To get around the difficulty, special registers of congenital anomalies, analagous to cancer registers, have sometimes been set up. These generally make use of a wide variety of information sources. An excellent example is the British Columbia Registry of Handicapped Children and Adults. One weakness of such undertakings, however, is that maintenance of the files is usually carried out manually. And yet, much of the information that is transmitted to a registry manually may exist also in machine readable form in the routine files of health records. Furthermore, these routine files often contain information about additional cases that are not known to the registries. Thus, the more source files that are tapped, the more complete becomes the ascertainment of cases, provided, of course, that the individuals are identified by name throughout so that the same person will not be counted more than once.

Data on this point have been obtained from a record linkage study in the province of Nova Scotia, based on their Central Registry of Handicapped Children on the provincial records of hospitalizations and deaths among infants (Table 1). It was found that although some of the cases appeared in all of the source files, the extent of the overlap was less than expected. When

TABLE 1

Cases of Congenital Anomalies Among 18,314 Children Born Alive In
Nova Scotia in 1964. (From Newcombe, 1969)[9]

Code	Anomaly	Total ascertained	Hosp. & Death	Registry
253	cretinism	3	3	1
295	hemophilia	1	—	1
325	mental deficiency	78	29	58
384	strabismus	66	—	67
389	blindness	—	—	1*
397	deaf-mutism	1	—	1
745	curvature of spine	1	1	1
748	clubfoot	57	24	47
750	monstrosity	10	10	—
751	spina bifida and meningocele	26	25	11
752	hydrocephalus	26	21	11
753	other c.m. of nervous system	14	11	3
754	c.m. of circulatory system	107	76	61
755	cleft palate and hare lip	40	33	33
756	c.m. of digestive system	141	138	6
757	c.m. of genito-urinary system	22	21	1
758	c.m. of bone and joint	50	31	25
759	other and unspecified c.m.	56	50	7
	multiple congenital anomalies	34	20	32
	Totals	733	493	367
	Percent	4.0	2.7	2.0

*Included among multiple anomalies in "Total ascertained" column.

all of the source records for a birth cohort were combined into a single integrated file of cases, 4 percent of children born alive were shown to have birth
defects, whereas the Registry alone was aware of only half this number, and
only two-thirds appeared among the combined hospital and death records.

The finding indicates that, if we are to know how many birth defects of the
various kinds there are, we will need to a) tap all usable files of source
records, b) ensure that individuals are adequately identified on their various
records, and c) automate the integration of the files so that it can be carried
out cheaply and quickly.

THE SEARCH FOR CAUSES

Having enumerated the congenital defects in a birth population, a next
logical question is "Why do they occur?" The quest for clues concerning
causal events of influences usually involves a search for unusual features in the
past histories of the mothers, either during their current pregnancies or at some
earlier time, or perhaps in the family histories of the mothers and fathers.

Substantial information about the relevant individual and family histories
may be extracted from routine files through the use of record linkage. I would
not wish to imply that all of the potentially important facts are recorded or
that *ad hoc* surveys will become unnecessary in the future. However, *ad hoc*
surveys of conventional design tend, for reasons of economy, to be limited in
size, and are therefore appropriate mainly for gathering those parts of the
histories that are not already recorded routinely in an accessible form. The
two approaches may, in fact, complement one another by each providing
different information about the same people. But, in general, only from the
routine records is it possible to compile follow-up histories for very large
populations and for whole geographic areas.

Our own experience in the search for causes relates to the Canadian
province of British Columbia, which has a current population of about two
million. Use has been made of records contained in their vital registration
system for the years 1946 through 1963, plus those of a special register of
handicapped children mentioned earlier. About 800,000 records of births
and parental marriages have been linked into sibship groupings, and records of
deaths and handicaps of children have been linked to the appropriate birth
records. Currently, methods are being developed to include also in the individual and family histories selected admission-discharge summaries for children
from a universal system of hospital insurance.

All of the above files exist already in machine-readable form. However, it
has sometimes been necessary to pay for a modest amount of special keypunching to enter into the machine-readable versions of the records more of

the personal identifying particulars contained in the original forms.

Using the vital registrations and the handicap register, it is possible to search for correlations between the risks of birth defects and the following variables:

— maternal age,
— birth order,
— paternal age,
— gestation,
— birth weight,
— race,
— season of birth,
— maternal fertility,
— child spacing, and
— prior births of stillborn, handicapped and dead siblings.

When records of hospitalizations of children have been added to the linked files, an improved picture of the sibship histories of morbidity will become available for correlation with the risks associated with particular pregnancies.

Examples of correlations already observed using the vital registrations and handicap register are given in Tables 2, 3 and 4. Maternal age, birth order and family history are all strongly correlated with the risks of various kinds of trouble for the newborn infants, observable at birth or shortly thereafter. Paternal age (independent of maternal) is also correlated with the occurrence of some birth anomalies but whether this represents a true cause-and-effect relationship is less certain.

The twin data (Table 4) are of special interest in relation to the definition of birth anomalies. Among like-sexed pairs of twins, approximately half of whom are genetically identical, there is a much stronger tendency than in the opposite sexed pairs for diseases that affect one twin to appear also in the other. Whether this concordance is due to a common heredity or to a common environment in a single amniotic sac need not concern us here since, in either case, the conditions involved must be congenital in origin. What is important is that the effect is not confined to the congenital malformations but is apparent in more than half of the broad categories of disease recognized by the International Classification. The evidence indicates that a much wider range of diseases of children is congenital in origin than is generally recognized. The phenomenon is worthy of more detailed study than we have been able to give it, but we happen to have the data solely because of the systematic manner in which we have linked the vital and health records for a large population.

No attempt has been made so far to explore exhaustively all of the possible associations between the risks of birth defects and the recorded variables

TABLE 2
Special Risks Associated With Parental Ages and Birth Orders
(From Newcombe, 1965)[6]

Code	Disease	Total Cases	Relative Risk	X^2 (DF = 1)
Children of older mothers (age 35–99 vs. 0–34)				
325.4	mongolism	191	7.68	172.6
351	cerebral palsy	215	1.84	11.6
754	c.m. of circulatory syst.	868	1.66	29.1
Children of older fathers (age 40–99 vs. 0–39)				
470-527	dis. of respiratory syst.	955	1.61	17.8
750-759	congenital malformations	1,727	1.28	9.1
135	other c.m. of nervous syst.	753	2.07	7.8
Children of higher birth orders (3rd and over vs. 1st and 2nd)				
001-138	infective and parasitic	146	1.76	9.9
384	strabismus	285	1.58	11.7
753	other c.m. of nervous syst.	175	1.84	12.1
762	postnatal asphyxia	773	1.70	39.2
Children of very young mothers (age 0–19 vs. 20–24)				
400-716	categories VI – XII	58	2.44	8.6
760	birth injury	72	2.19	9.6
762	postnatal asphyxia	413	1.66	15.4
Firstborn children (vs. 2nd)				
760-776	diseases of early infancy	58	2.16	10.6
760	birth injury	123	1.80	9.1

Note: Maternal age effects above have birth order effects removed and *vice versa*, and paternal age effects have maternal age effects removed.

TABLE 3

Special Risks Associated With Diseases of Previously Born Brothers and Sisters
(From Newcombe, 1966) [7]

Code	Disease Category	Cases in birth population*	Cases in later sibs/ unaffected	Relative risk
750	monstrosity	41	3/21	707.2
389	blindness	53	2/42	182.4
757	congenital malformation of genito-urinary system	140	3/57	76.3
753	other c.m. of nervous system	168	4/67	72.1
384	strabismus	286	10/171	41.5
766	immaturity	1,089	105/467	41.1
762	postnatal asphyxia	742	35/355	27.0
758	congenital malformation of bone	168	1/64	18.9
325	mental deficiency	568	12/286	15.0
755	cleft palate and lip	341	3/132	13.5
748	clubfoot	408	5/194	12.8
759	other congenital malformations	200	1/99	10.3
760	birth injury	219	1/125	7.8
754	congenital malformation of circulatory system	837	7/390	4.4

*Versus 202,968 unaffected.

TABLE 4

Special Risks Associated With Diseases of Co-twins of Like and Opposite Sex
(From Newcombe, 1968) [8]

Code	Disease Category	Concordant/discordant like	opposite	Ratio like/ opposite
001-138	infective and parasitic	1/2	0/2	
140-239	neoplasms	0/6	0/5	
240-289	allergic, endocrine, etc.	0/1	0/2	
290-299	blood forming organs	0/0	0/0	
300-326	mental, psychoneurotic, etc.	4/13	0/6	
330-398	nervous system and sense organs	3/17	0/7	
400-468	circulatory system	0/0	0/0	
470-527	respiratory system	1/16	0/7	
530-587	digestive system	1/5	0/6	
590-637	genito-urinary system	0/1	0/0	
690-716	skin and cellular tissue	0/0	0/0	
729-749	bones and organs of movement	2/7	0/7	
750-759	congenital malformations	4/44	0/14	
780-795	symptoms and ill-defined	0/0	0/1	
800-999	accidents, etc.	1/2	0/2	
Y30-Y39	stillbirths, all causes	21/61	1/29	
- -	other (except 760-776)	1/209	0/99	
	combined	39/384	1/182	18.5
760-776	diseases of early infancy	68/88	32/34	0.8

listed earlier. There would be no major obstacle, however, to using the linked files in such a manner.

THE NATURAL HISTORY OF THE DISEASES

A further question related to the magnitude of the harm caused by the various birth defects. Counts of the numbers of affected individuals alone are a poor measure of the total harm. What is needed is information about the extent of the effects which the conditions have on the lives of these people from birth onward or, in other words, statistics on the natural histories of the diseases. In the past, these have been readily obtainable only for those individuals who died early because of the conditions or remained permanently in institutions. For the defects that do not remove the affected individuals from society, such statistics would be even more important but they have been much less readily obtainable by any conventional method.

To assess the total impact, one would wish to know the extents to which the affected individuals differ from others, for example:
— their needs for hospital services,
— their successes in school,
— their abilities to obtain employment,
— the likelihood of marriage,
— the numbers of offspring they produce, and
— the ages at which they eventually die.

All such information is, in fact, recorded routinely in a form that identifies it with the individuals concerned. In Canada at least, the files are largely centralized and mechanized. If we want to know more about the lifetime impact of the birth defects, one way to find out would be to extend the principle of record linkage to include not only the health related records but those pertaining to the economic and social characteristics of the individuals as well.

I will not belabor this further point, because I feel we should first tidy up the health records so as to make full use of them. But the possibility of such an extension exists, and the technical difficulties are not as great as one might suppose.

THE SUCCESSES OF TREATMENTS

Even the essentially medical problem of assessing the successes of particular methods of treatment and of management involves follow-up of individuals. Where only short periods of observation are needed, current methods of follow-up may be adequate. But what if the assessments ought correctly to be in terms of the maintenance of improvements over the lifetimes of the affected individuals? For example, what are (or what will be) the relevant lifetime statistics on children treated for cystic fibrosis, galactosemia, tyrosinemia, phenylketonuria, Wilson's disease, cretinism, juvenile diabetes and cerebral palsy of various degrees of severity? To what extents do the standard methods of treatment, when applied early, normalize the patterns of their lives ten, twenty or thirty years later?

Past experience has shown that conventional methods of follow-up are suitable for the purposes of such long term studies only as applied to small numbers of cases. It follows that we might hope to be better guided in the choice between alternative methods of treatment, where alternatives exist, if use could be made of existing routine documentation of relevant events throughout the lives of much larger numbers of affected individuals.

The vital records systems of most countries can be made to yield life tables for selected individuals, and the hospital insurance records of some areas, of which Canada is one, are capable of yielding histories of repeat hospitalizations. These, in turn, would permit comparisons on the basis of the methods of treatment and management, the stages at which treatment was commenced, and so on.

In practice, where large routine files are employed for follow-up using computer methods, it is most efficient to follow all known cases of all diseases of interest in the whole area represented by the files. The reason for this is that the cost of scanning the large files tends to be a constant, regardless of the number of persons being followed.

THE COST OF FAILURES

In a similar fashion, and using the same approach, we might ask the question, "What is the cost to society and to the individual of failures to prevent the occurrences of various birth defects, or to detect and treat them early enough?" Such a question may be answered statistically in a number of ways, for example, in terms of:
  — the resulting additional utilization of hospital facilities,
  — losses of years of schooling,
  — losses of opportunities for productive employment, and
  — the probable total economic loss to society arising out of these more specific consequences.

The detailed answers to such questions might or might not contain surprises. But, in either case, the results would provide a sounder basis for setting priorities in the prevention, detection, management and treatment of congenital defects. They should also provide some measure of the economic benefits to society to be expected from investments in relevant public health programs, quite apart from the usual humanitarian considerations.

It is worth mentioning, in this connection, that Canada possesses a centralized file of unemployment insurance records, in machine-readable form, in which the cumulative work histories of a continuing 5 percent sample of the labor force are represented by annual punch cards containing details of occupations, industries and geographic locations, together with the social insurance numbers and surnames of the individuals concerned.

There is also a move in this country, sponsored by the provincial ministers of education, to identify children by social insurance numbers from age 14 or grade 7 onward so their educational careers may be followed throughout the school system and into the labor force, regardless of the migrations of the pupils between schools. As emphasized earlier, however, experience with the proposed kind of follow-up is needed first, with the health records systems, before serious consideration is given to the extensive use of other large files.

THE METHODS OF FOLLOW-UP

All of the possibilities discussed so far hinge on the technical feasibility and cost of manipulating very large files of vital records and hospital records for the purpose of arranging them into groups representing the health histories of individual people and families. The prime requirement is that the personal identifying information contained in the records be sufficient to distinguish one person from another.

In the case of the vital records, which are legal documents, the identifying information is quite adequate for the purpose of linkage. Moreover, much of it finds its way routinely into the machine-readable versions of the records for the purpose of preparing alphabetic indexes of births, deaths and marriages so that registry office staff can locate any record in their files in order to issue certificates as required by the public. In both Canada and the United States such indexes are derived from punch cards that contain the relevant names, dates and places. In Canada, in recent years, some additional family identifying information has been entered into these index cards, in the form of the maiden surname of the mother of a newborn child and a deceased individual, together with the initials, ages and birthplace codes for the parental couples. This makes possible a matching of the birth records with the parental marriage records and with the birth records of brothers and sisters into sibship groupings, and a matching of death records with the birth records for the deceased individuals.

A file of some 800,000 family-linked vital records for the province of British Columbia has been built up covering the period 1946 through 1963,

105

and records of handicapped children have been integrated into this linked file.

In hospital admission-discharge records, the personal identifying information is less specific. In Canada, although such records are standardized within all provinces, there is little uniformity between provinces with respect to the identifying particulars. For purposes of follow-up, one would like to have the birth name, birth date and birth place of each hospitalized person. Only one Canadian province (Nova Scotia) asks for all three on its forms, and the other provinces ask for only one of the three items (see Table 5).

The British Columbia hospital insurance records, fortunately for our own work, contain two of the items, birth name and birth data. For young children, a majority of whom are born in the province anyway, this is sufficient to permit linkage of the hospital records with the appropriate birth records. Currently, Miss Martha Smith of the Chalk River Nuclear Laboratories is developing the computer methods with which to link some 200,000 hospital records for children with congenital and other diseases, discharged over a ten year period, to one another in individual histories of repeated hospitalization, and to the birth records and family histories.

The task of matching two or more records pertaining to the same individual is complicated by frequent inaccuracies in the names and other details of identification. To be efficient, the computer programs must therefore simulate the subjective judgment of a human filing clerk who is assigned a similar task. This implies attaching some sort of "weight" to each agreement and disagreement of the various identifying particulars on two records that are being compared. For example, agreement of the initial Z will carry more weight than agreement of the initial J, simply because it is less common. Similarly, a difference in birth date will carry more negative weight as indicating a non-linkage than would a difference in the address, since changes of address are fairly common in comparison with errors in birth date. Considerable effort has been spent on the development of an adequate mathematical and empirical basis for this approach.[1]

The accuracy with which the computer links the records is at least as high as that of a human filing clerk, and the computer has the added advantage that it can indicate in numerical form the degree of certainty or uncertainty concerning a linkage or a failure to link.

The linkage operation proper is also both fast and cheap. Only the process of preparing the files for linkage, where the records are not initially designed for the purpose, has proved laborious and time consuming. In one of our early tests approximately 98.4 percent of potentially linkable birth and marriage

TABLE 5

Identifying Information Contained in the Hospital Admission-Discharge
Summaries for the Different Provincial Insurance Schemes in Canada
(From Newcombe, 1970)[10]

Province	Maiden name	Birth date	Birth place
Newfoundland	−	+	−
Prince Edward Island	+	+	−
Nova Scotia	+	+	+
New Brunswick	−	+	+
Quebec	−	−	−
Ontario	−	−	+
Manitoba	−	+	−
Saskatchewan	−	+	−
Alberta	−	−	−
British Columbia	+	+	−
Northwest Territories	+	+	−

Based on 1968 forms for Alberta and 1969 forms for all other provinces.

records were correctly linked by computer, with an admixture of only 2 false linkages per thousand genuine. The linkages were carried out at a rate of 2,300 incoming birth records per minute and a unit cost less than the value of the individual blank punch cards.

At this point, I should like to make a plea for greater uniformity in the manner in which people are identified in their medical and other personal records, and for greater specificity of the identifying particulars requested on the forms. If one needs to know to whom a record refers, it is obviously not sufficient to be told just that the patient's name is Mary Smith and that she is age 25. At least three basic items should be on all forms, namely:
- birth date,
- birth place, and
- birth name.

In other words, the patient should be asked, "When were you born? Where were you born? And, what did they call you when you were born?" to ensure that there will be no confusion later over which person the record refers to.

THE PROBLEM OF DATA SOURCES

You may wonder, perhaps, if the whole proposal to link such diverse and bulky files into cradle-to-grave histories, and even into family histories, is just an elaborate piece of wishful thinking. Let us therefore attempt to assess realistically the magnitudes of some of the obstacles.

Technical feasibility of the linkage process is not the major problem. We have already carried out many such linkages so there is no doubt that they can be achieved rapidly and cheaply, and that the information sought can be extracted in a useful form.

The greatest difficulty arises because of the amount of time and effort that must be spent in order to arrange with the various custodians of the source files for the use of the records, under conditions acceptable to the responsible agencies and compatible with the requirements for maintaining the confidentiality of personal information. Most of the organizational and jurisdictional problems are solvable, but few people are as yet inclined, or in a position, to make the necessary investment of time and effort.

In this connection, I would like to pay tribute to the success of Dr. Donald Acheson and his successor, Dr. John Baldwin, in organizing an on-going record linkage facility in the Oxford Hospital Region in Britain[2,3] and to the sophisticated groundwork for such a scheme carried out by Professor Eric Cheeseman and his colleagues in Northern Ireland.[4]

There are also obstacles that arise because of the potential users themselves.

If custodians of the records occasionally take a parochial view of their responsibilities, so also do some of the potential users of the data. We may remind ourselves that the important units are not the agencies themselves, but the sick people whom the agencies were set up to serve. Similarly, those investigators who are interested in a particular category of disease, such as the birth defects, should not forget that the linked files are capable of answering similar questions with respect to other categories of disease, such as cancer.

The point is important when costs are considered, because the same manipulations of the files may be made to serve a multiplicity of quite diverse purposes without any great increase in effort and computer time. Thus, rather in the fashion that one might justify the purchase of, let us say an electron microscope, on the grounds of a multiplicity of uses to which it can be put, so one must justify the use of a record linkage facility in terms of the data it will make available concerning a wide range of diseases. The tool will not come into existence if its potential users are too parochial in their outlook and think only of their own specialties. Some collaborative organizational effort among various kinds of potential users is essential if a record linkage facility is to be established, and is to gain stability and permanence on the basis of its merits. I would suggest that such collaboration might well be established between those interested in teratogenesis, carcino-genesis and mutagenesis.

One further obstacle to such an undertaking is the sheer physical size of the accumulated files themselves. Even when stored on magnetic tape, the numbers of records required for a record linkage facility covering a population numbering in the tens of millions or more could be exceedingly bulky. The problem is fortunately solvable, and there are now a number of devices which will store as much as 10^{12} bits of information (equivalent to a thousand million records of the size used in our own work). Most of such devices use laser technology to write optically on photosensitive materials. Unlike magnetic fields, laser beams can be focused onto spots not much larger than a wavelength of light. In practice, the size of the individual "bits" may be in the vicinity of 5 microns, and the result is an increase in storage density as great as 100-fold or more.

One such defice, the UNICON 690-212 laser mass memory system produced by Precision Instrument Company, is currently being used by Standard Oil (Indiana) to store seismic findings, and another unit of the same kind is attached to the Illiac IV computer at the University of Illinois. The device is said to have a maximum random access time of 8 seconds, a transfer rate of 4 megabits per second, and to store information at a cost of 0.0001 cents per bit or 0.1 cent for a 1000-bit record.[5] Information on the perform-ance of such equipment is hard to obtain, but in view of the growing demand, it seems unlikely that more general use of compact mass storage will be long delayed.

In fact, none of the obstacles to record linkage mentioned above would seem to constitute a valid reason for failing to develop the existing collective documentation, so that one can study the sequences of major events in the lives of large numbers of people, rather than just the individual episodes in isolation from one another.

CONCLUSION

Is there really any other way of getting the information that this approach can yield, and of getting it systematically and in similar quantities?

Ad hoc surveys, necessary as they may be for many purposes, are by their nature limited in size and continuity. These characteristics, in turn, frequently limit the precision and the sensitivity of detection of such conventional approaches. I would propose that there is no competing alternative to record linkage where large quantities of follow-up data are required, except that of remaining in ignorance on many questions that are in need of answers. This would seem a shame where the questions are important and the answers remain locked in files that have already been accumulated at considerable cost for other purposes, and which are likely to be discarded if not further used.

REFERENCES

1. H.B. Newcombe, *Amer. J. Hum. Genet. 19,* 335, 1967.

2. E.D. Acheson, *in* Record Linkage in Medicine, E.D. Acheson (Ed.), E. and S. Livingston Ltd., Edinburgh, p. 40, 1967.

3. J.A. Baldwin and L.E. Gill, *in* Research Report No. 3, Oxford University Unit of Clinical Epidemiology and Oxford Regional Hospital Board.

4. E.A. Cheeseman, *in* Report No. RLU 3, Department of Medical Statistics, the Queen's University of Belfast, Belfast, 1971.

5. J.F. Terdiman, *Computers and Biological Research 3,* 528, 1970.

6. H.B. Newcombe, *Eugenics Review 57,* 109, 1965.

7. H.B. Newcombe, *Brit. J. Prev. and Soc. Med. 20,* 49, 1966.

8. H.B. Newcombe, *in* Record Linkage in Medicine, E.D. Acheson (Ed.), E. and S. Livingston Ltd., Edinburgh, p. 7, 1968.

9.   H.B. Newcombe, *Brit. J. Prev. and Soc. Med. 23,* 226, 1969.

10. H.B. Newcombe, *Medical Care 8,* 209, 1970.

DISCUSSION

DR. LILIENFELD: Dr. Valadian, did your reproductive index include a complete range of reproductive problems. For example, did it include eclampsia, pre-eclampsia and albuminuria? Secondly, how did you arrive at the age breakdown which you used for your analysis? Was the subdivision made according to an *a priori* hypothesis?

DR. VALADIAN: The reproductive index was developed from a list which included a complete range of complications of pregnancy including the most slight through the most severe. In answer to the second part of your question, we examined each possible relationship by subdividing the ages into infancy, preschool, etc.

DR. LILIENFELD: Dr. Janerich, in examining the possible causes of each peak, you neglected to discuss the major peak which occurred in these malformations during the early 1900's in Providence. Secondly, I think your analysis is most interesting and it suggests that New York State would be an excellent place to begin a study of young mothers of anencephalic children in order to search for the possible effects of early environmental exposures.

DR. JANERICH: The early peak in the Providence data is difficult to evaluate. The numbers are quite small during that period and there is a large difference between the rates in Providence and Boston. The difference between the hospitals may be a function of basic socio-economic factors in these populations. Of course, we must consider the possibility that each peak represents a separate epidemic event. As far as studies on young mothers, we are proceeding with such studies. In addition, we are suggesting that congenital malformation monitoring programs include more background information from the parent's health history.

DR. NANCE: I think an important factor which is often neglected is the genetic-environmental interaction. This came out in Dr. Fraser's data where it is clear that the influence of diet depends upon the genotype. I differ to some extent with one of Dr. Janerich's statements. I believe that if we can identify genotypes in which there is a high risk, that there is some hope for prevention through prenatal detection. The underlying mechanisms of genetic-environmental interactions need not be complex and multifactorial. We certainly have an excellent example in the development of hemolytic anemia in individuals with G6PD deficiency. This is a highly specific genetic-environmental interaction that has a simple genetic basis.

DR. JANERICH: I agree with your observation, Dr. Nance, and that is why I suggested that it would be wise to incorporate more information on parental factors into our congenital malformations monitoring programs. This type of information might provide us with some valuable clues to genetic-environmental interactions. But at the present time, the polygenic concept of causation has provided very little help in the development of preventive measures.

KENNETH P. JOHNSON: Dr. Janerich, there is one other epidemic to consider. Between 1920 and 1945 there was an epidemic of *Encephalitis lethargica*, or von Economos disease, which we recognize as having produced postencephalitic Parkinson's disease. The person affected had a delayed central nervous system disease fifteen to twenty years later. Whether there could be some effect on some other system in the maternal host besides the nervous system, no one has ever considered.

DR. JANERICH: I am aware of that epidemic. I think Poskanzer proposed the possible cohort mechanisms. It is an interesting situation, and it seems to be worth considering the possibility that other host systems may have been permanently affected.

MELITA GESCHE (New York State Department of Health, Albany, New York): Dr. Valadian, do you know of any study where the intake of protein in the four years, from eight to twelve years of age, was ascertained by recall rather than by direct longitudinal observation? I am wondering if it could be done in a different population and thereby shorten the whole study. For instance, in the so-called developing countries where you could, by recall and taboos in certain villages, find out what the intake has been in the four years preceding menarche. Since they start their reproduction rather early, their post-menarche period might also be a relatively shorter one than the ones that appear when women start having their children rather late in life.

DR. VALADIAN: There are other longitudinal studies both in the United States and abroad, namely in London, Stockholm, Zurich and Brussels. These studies were started after 1949. Their subjects are now in the adolescent age period so it is early for us to get any supporting data from those studies. As far as the other studies in the United States, we are trying to pool our data to obtain a larger number with which to test a hypothesis. As far as going into an area and gathering retrospective information, it is difficult to base conclusions on that type of information. I understand there is a population in Northern Japan, where, at a given time in a group of orphanages, the city fathers made a sudden change in the food served to the children. We are trying to see if we can determine whether the girls who experienced that change during their early adolescent period, are having any different reproductive experience than the girls who were affected by the dietary change before that age.

PHILIP SPIERS (National Institutes of Health, Bethesda, Maryland): If it is reasonable to suppose that the protein intake varies with socio-economic status, does it not follow that the variation in reproduction performance which you have observed may be related to some other agent associated with socio-economic status?

DR. VALADIAN: The group was quite homogenous in terms of socio-economic status. The patients were selected by Dr. Stuart in 1930, from the Boston Lying-In Hospital's Prenatal Clinic. In the 1930's, people who were poor were going to the Boston City Hospital because they could not afford private care. In addition, right from the start of the study, they had social workers visiting the homes and assessing the home situation. Dr. Stuart wanted to have a group that was homogeneous both racially and ethnically. He selected young families (parents) that were born in the United States but were of North European descent. A third condition was that the fathers would be reasonably sure to remain around Boston for at least six years. Therefore, he selected families with men who had steady occupations. There were a lot of policemen, small grocery store owners, etc. So, we have the data which the social workers were bringing in for describing these families. They were mostly of the low middle income group.

STEVEN PAUKER (Massachusetts General Hospital, Boston, Massachusetts): Dr. Valadian, I have a question about the accuracy of your dietary histories. Over the seven or eight years before menarche your data shows that the protein intake went up only about 20 to 40 percent, while through these age ranges we would expect body weight to increase by 100 percent.

DR. VALADIAN: In terms of the adequacy of the dietary histories, the reliability was tested by Dr. Reed in 1959. The fact that Mrs. Burke had developed the method and had carried all dietary histories herself, is a safeguard. I admit that dietary histories are certainly subject to errors. The safeguard is the continuity of the same interviewer and the fact that the subjects become accustomed to answering the questions, observing and become better information sources. If you go into a population at large and take a dietary history, there is more chance of error than if you are dealing with a stable group that is being interviewed year after year.

MRS. ROSALIE GREEN: Dr. Janerich, the three areas that you discussed were primarily in the Northeast. Anencephaly, in particular, has been shown to be concentrated most frequently in England, going from south to north and seems to disappear across the European continent toward Asia. I've always questioned measurements on anencephaly in Asia. Have you compared this type of data with the southern part of the United States which has a high concentration of British descendants and also correlated it with the immigration or country of origin of the people who were affected by this disease?

DR. JANERICH: I am afraid the status of the data on these malformations is not such that large-scale studies of that type can be attempted. I think Doctors MacMahon and Yen have contributed a key piece of information by assembling the longitudinal data set which showed that a giant epidemic of anencephaly and spina bifida had occurred during the early part of the century. I think their effort will turn out to be a significant step forward in understanding the etiology of these malformations. Also, I do agree with you that the data which we have available from Asia is of questionable quality.

WILLIAM ZWARTJEN (Massachusetts General Hospital, Boston, Massachusetts): Dr. Valadian, I have another question about your data. You gave the protein intake, in grams, for each person. I wonder how this relates to grams per kilogram of body weight since I think the intake protein would vary by the size of the person.

DR. VALADIAN: We have also worked that out but I didn't bring those data with me and I don't have the answer to that, at hand.

SECTION III

SECTION III

TRENDS IN SURVEILLANCE OF CONGENITAL MALFORMATIONS

J. William Flynt, Jr.

Speakers at the Birth Defects Institute Symposium held in 1970 discussed in detail surveillance of a number of birth defects to detect the introduction of environmental teratogens or mutagens in the population.[1] The purpose of this paper is to consider the present status of congenital malformation surveillance in this country and to deal particularly with monitoring of data for changes in frequency.

The term "surveillance" has been widely used in infectious disease epidemiology to mean a continued watchfulness over the distribution and changes in incidence of a disease through systematic collection and evaluation of data. An integral part of such activities is the regular reporting of basic data with interpretation to contributors and to others who need to know.[2] In this context the term "surveillance" carries a sense of immediacy about reporting and analysis of data. "Surveillance" has also been applied to malformations, but its use has been broader and frequently means data collection analysis without any sense of immediacy or provision for returning the data to those who have contributed. In a survey of State Crippled Children's and Maternal and Child Health directors in 1965, 19 states and 24 cities with over 100,000 population were using birth certificates for epidemiologic surveillance. However, of the 33 who noted the frequency with which their data were reviewed, only 12 reported reviews at monthly or quarterly intervals. The other 21 examined their data annually or at irregular intervals.[3]

PURPOSES OF MALFORMATION SURVEILLANCE

The various purposes for which malformation data have been collected may account for the broader use of the term "surveillance". Participants in a recent WHO consultation defined 6 purposes of malformation surveillance:

> Monitoring
> Epidemiologic Studies
> Registries
> Detection of New Syndromes
> Medical and Lay Education
> Public Relations

119

Each purpose has somewhat different requirements for the type and quality of data needed, the sources of such data and the speed of reporting and analyses required.

Monitoring

Monitoring of malformations is used more frequently to convey the sense of immediacy that is needed when looking for changes in malformation incidence or altered patterns that environmental agents might cause. This use requires prompt case reporting and data analysis (within 1−2 months of birth) and will focus less on complete case ascertainment and more on prompt reporting. For monitoring purposes, a variety of data sources can be used including vital records, special studies or registries, hospital discharge summaries, and clinical records of specialty centers. Although these sources may contain biases and inaccuracies, they nevertheless are still useful since the concern is with changes over time and these will be apparent as long as the biases of the data source remain relatively constant.

The use of monitoring as a distinct purpose for surveillance of malformations seems warranted on 2 accounts. It focuses clearly on the need for prompt case detection and immediate data review, and it avoids unpleasant overtones of invading personal privacy that the term surveillance sometimes brings.

Epidemiologic Studies

Data collected for descriptive epidemiologic studies are most commonly used to characterize racial, sexual, maternal age and seasonal differences associated with malformations and to define particular high or low incidence population groups. Such studies require sizable populations and several data sources to ensure complete case ascertainment. In such instances, complete reporting is of primary concern, and the delay between the birth of the infant and the report of a malformation may be of little consequence, since data analysis is generally deferred until enough cases are obtained, sometimes years after the infants birth.

Registries

Malformation registries are most commonly used for planning, delivering and evaluating medical care or to provide data for genetic or other studies that require regular family followup. The chief concerns of surveillance for a registry may be complete ascertainment and establishing procedures for maintaining contact with the families. In these circumstances, prompt reporting is of secondary importance except for those whose purpose it is to provide care to the infant or family.

Detection of New Syndromes

Malformation surveillance to detect new syndromes or associations of malformations is a specialized use of surveillance that depends on obtaining detailed and uniform clinical information. Particular attention must be given to standard examinations of the infants, with careful documentation and uniform description of all defects. Attention to such detail can be time consuming and restrict the number of newborns studied. Such approaches are often best handled in a few hospitals or circumstances where observer variability can be controlled. In such circumstances, speed of reporting becomes secondary to accuracy and completeness, and data analysis may also be deferred for considerable periods of time. Källen and Winberg have shown that this need not always be the case; they used monitored data from the Swedish national malformation register to identify a new syndrome.[4,5]

Education and Public Relations

These last 2 purposes are ancillary services that most any surveillance program could provide. Physicians and the general public often need information about sources and availability of health care, genetic counselling and diagnostic services. Surveillance programs can serve as a focal point for providing such information. Increasing public concern with environmental agents and their roles in the etiology of malformations can be answered only with accurate data, readily accessible to those who need to know.

MALFORMATION MONITORING IN THE UNITED STATES

Surveillance for the purpose of monitoring has developed slowly in this country. The first such program began at the New York State Health Department in May 1962, 6 months after the removal of thalidomide from the British market; Milham began reviewing birth records from upstate New York at monthly intervals looking for trends or clusters of defects that might reflect environmental factors.[6] Other states and some cities appear also to have instituted similar measures, for in 1965 the survey by Dr. Helen Wallace found that some 43 states and cities were using birth certificates for epidemiologic surveillance.[3] However, over 60% of the areas examined their data so infrequently that increases could have continued for several months before detection. At present 4 surveillance programs in this country monitor malformation data and regularly exchange information on suspicious occurrences (Table 1). A fifth program, located in Los Angeles, California, also monitored data until its termination in October 1972.[7] The remaining 4 programs compile data on roughly 275,000 births a year, or approximately 8% of the nation's total. The programs differ considerably in the number of newborns included, ranging from

TABLE 1

Current Malformation Surveillance and Monitoring Programs
in the United States

Location	Year Started	Geographic Area	Number of Births	Data Sources[1]
Albany, N.Y.	1962	Upstate New York	180,000	V. R.
Atlanta, Ga.	1967	5 counties	30,000	H.R.,V.R.
Olympia, Wash.	1968	Washington	54,000	V. R.
Los Angeles, Calif.[2]	1969	8 hospitals	25,000	H.R.,V.R.
Jacksonville, Fla.	1971	6 counties	12,000	H.R.,V.R.

[1]V.R. = Vital Records
 H.R. = Hospital Records

[2]Terminated October 31, 1972

12,000 to 180,000 births, and in geographic coverage. These programs also differ in the sources of data used for surveillance; Washington and New York use vital records only, while these and hospital records are used for surveillance in Atlanta and Florida.

The Center for Disease Control is directly involved in the Atlanta and Florida surveillance programs. Florida surveillance is funded by the Florida Regional Medical Program and operated by the Division of Health of the Florida Department of Health and Rehabilitative Services in a 6-county region of northeast Florida. Reports of malformed infants under age 7 days are provided voluntarily by medical record librarians in all area hospitals who abstract onto precoded forms epidemiologic data for affected infants discharged from their hospitals. These forms are sent monthly to CDC for keypunching and computer processing of the data, which are then returned to the state for its use.

Surveillance in Atlanta is conducted by the staff of the Metropolitan Atlanta Congenital Defects Program, a cooperative project of the Center for Disease Control, the Georgia Mental Health Institute, and the Emory University School of Medicine.[8] The staff regularly visit nurseries, obstetrical units and medical record rooms of each hospital in the 5-county metropolitan area to identify infants under age 1 year born with malformations. Information on these infants is obtained from hospital records and abstracted onto precoded forms for data processing.

A bimonthly report prepared and distributed by CDC contains surveillance data from Atlanta and northeast Florida and brief reports of epidemiologic studies, summaries of unusual increases in incidence or results of other investigations. These reports are available to all who assist in providing the data and others with an interest in or need for such information.

A COMPUTER MONITORING SYSTEM

Monitoring should ensure that each defect category is reviewed regularly and systematically to identify sudden increases in incidence and more gradual, but continued upward trends. Marked increases and changes in the occurrence of rare anomalies may be noted by inspection of the data, but gradual increases of even marked changes could be overlooked among the number of defects — some 130 different categories in the ICDA — which are scrutinized. To assist in these efforts we have developed and used since April 1971 a computerized statistical monitoring system (Table 2).

In the system, data for 1968–1970 are used as baseline incidence rates with which to calculate for each defect an expected number of cases [E (C)] for 1, 2, 4, 6, 12–month, and cumulative periods. These expected numbers are

TABLE 2

Sample Format of Congenital Malformation Statistical Monitoring System

Defect Category 490

Incidence Rate is 0.39

Observation Period

Month & Year	1–Month			2–Month			4–Month			6–Month			12–Month			Cumulative*		
	CE	(C)	IND	CE	(C)	IND	CE	(C)	IND	CE	(C)	IND	CE	(C)	IND	CE	(C)	IND
8/72	0.	0.	0	0.	2.	0	1.	4.	0	3.	5.	0	16.	11.	0	55.	42.	0
7/72	0.	0.	0	0.	2.	0	2.	4.	0	5.	5.	0	18.	11.	0	55.	41.	0
6/72	0.	0.	0	1.	2.	0	3.	4.	0	7.	5.	0	21.	11.	2	55.	40.	0
5/72	0.	0.	0	2.	2.	0	5.	4.	0	8.	5.	0	23.	11.	4	55.	39.	1

*Extends from January 1, 1969.

124

then compared with the observed cases (C), and whenever case occurrence exceeds the expected by 2 standard deviations, using the Poisson distribution, the defect is listed on a computer printout. The number of observed cases that exceed the 2 standard deviation level are also displayed (IND), Comparisons are made for the current reporting month and also for the 3 preceding months in order that late reported cases may appear in the analysis.

Since the inception of the monitoring system, a total of 23 defects have shown increases significant at the 0.01 level. Changes in statistical sensitivity would alter the number of defects listed, but the present load of 0—2 new defects a month noted by the monitoring has proved manageable in our situation.

No environmental causes have been identified to explain these increases. Three defects noted by the monitoring system are of particular interest (Table 2). An increase in the incidence of cleft palate was first noted in May 1971; this continued throughout the remainder of the year. Incidence rates in 1971 rose over 2-fold higher than those in 1968—1970 but have subsequently returned to earlier levels. The 1971 cases occurred throughout the year and without any geographic localization. No changes in race or sex distributions were noted, and no other defects were associated in the patients with cleft palates. Interviews of the mothers of these affected infants yielded no evidence of common associations nor exposures to infectious agents or drugs.

The incidence of polydactyly has risen since surveillance began in 1968, from 3.54 per 1,000 total births to 4.17 and 4.06 per 1,000 in 1971 and 1972, respectively. The increase was first noted by the monitoring system in July 1971 and can be attributed to changes in case reporting and composition of the population. A slight rise in incidence over this period occurred among blacks; white races have remained essentially level. The substantial rise in total rates resulted from the higher black rates and an increase over these years in the proportion of black births from 27% in 1968 to 30% in 1971. Because of these findings no further investigation of the increase seemed necessary.

A modest increase occurred in 1971 in the incidence of all cases with reduction deformities (Table 3). A transient increase in upper limb deformities occurred in the summer of 1971 and a more sustained increase in lower extremity reduction-type deformities was noted by the monitoring system in November 1971. Rates for lower limb deformities were approximately 2 times higher in 1971 than during the 1968—1971 base period. These increases, considered in the light of recent reports from Canada[9] and Australia[10] of other increases or unusual associations with reduction deformities, seemed worthy of special attention. Cases in Atlanta ranged from missing digits to losses of major portions of one or more extremity. No associations with other defects were present. Some of the mothers were interviewed regarding their ingestion

TABLE 3

Annual Incidence Rates[*] of Selected Malformations, Metropolitan Atlanta

January 1, 1968 — October 31, 1972

Defect	1968	1969	1970	1971	1972
Cleft palate	0.37	0.36	0.43	0.84	0.48
Polydactyly	3.54	3.38	3.78	4.17	4.06
Reduction deformities					
Upper	0.75	0.47	0.50	0.56	0.35
Lower	0.30	0.25	0.37	0.63	0.39
Total[**]	0.89	0.68	0.76	1.01	0.74

[*] Per 1,000 total births

[**] Cases with upper and/or lower extremity reduction deformities

of tricyclic antidepressants, and no link between cases and these drugs were found. [11]

DISCUSSION

To develop intensive surveillance to collect data for monitoring only is probably unwise because of costs and the infrequency with which environmental associations are apt to be detected. A more desirable approach would be to ensure that available malformation data and those collected for other purposes are monitored. Vital records, despite their deficiencies, offer one source of available data. Health data services, such as those operated by the Commission on Professional and Hospital Activities and member organizations of the American Association of Health Data Systems, already collect information on a substantial number of the nation's births that might well be used for monitoring.

Other sources of data may emerge as surveillance programs develop to provide information for special epidemiologic studies, to measure the effectiveness of preventive measures on genetic disease, and to improve care for the family and infant with a malformation. Wherever such programs develop, provisions should be included for monitoring of the data collected.

Monitoring is one way to look for environmental causes of malformations, but suspicions of such causes will come also from other quarters. Clinical observations, such as those that led to the recognition of the effects of rubella and thalidomide, will provide leads about environmental factors. Other leads will come from epidemiological and laboratory investigations. Such ideas may need urgent testing on other populations; for example, surveillance programs with provisions for prompt review and use of data.

There need be no arguments about the most desirable approach to identifying environmental teratogens. We should use whatever sources are available, evaluating and comparing their usefulness with the understanding that each may make its contribution to detecting environmental causes of birth defects.

REFERENCES

1. E.B. Hook, D.T. Janerich and I.H. Porter (Eds.), *in* Monitoring, Birth Defects and Environment, The Problem of Surveillance, Academic Press, New York, 1971.

2. A.D. Langmuir, *New Engl. J. Med. 268,* 182, 1963.

3. H.M. Wallace and S. T. Fisher, *Pub. Health Rep. 81,* 631, 1966.

4. B. Källen and J. Winberg, *Pediatrics 44,* 410, 1969.

5. B. Källen and J. Winberg, *Pediatrics 41,* 765, 1969.

6. S. Milham, Jr., *Pub. Health Rep. 78,* 448, 1963.

7. A.J. Ebbin and M.G. Wilson, *in* Fetal Sequelae of Rubella Immunization and Birth Defects Program in Los Angeles County in loc. cit (ref. 1), P. 159.

8. J.W. Flynt, A.J. Ebbin, G.P. Oakley, A. Falek and C.W. Heath, Metropolitan Atlanta Congenital Defects Program in loc. cit (ref. 1), p. 155.

9. P. Banister, *Canad. Med. Assoc. J. 103,* 446, 1970.

10. W.G. McBride, *Med. J. Australia 1,* 492, 1972.

11. G.S. Rachelefsky, J.W. Flynt, A.J. Ebbin and M.G. Wilson, *Lancet 1,* 838, 1972.

CONGENITAL RUBELLA:
THE INDIRECT APPROACH TO PREVENTION

Alan R. Hinman

Rubella has been described since early in the eighteenth century and since 1881 it has been agreed that it is a distinct illness. Until 1941 it was regarded as an extremely benign childhood disease with very few complications, although it had been noted that arthralgia was fairly common especially in adults.

In 1941, Gregg reported, from Australia, the occurrence of congenital cataracts, retinopathy and congenital heart disease in infants born of women who had had rubella during pregnancy. Since 1941 many other supportive data have been accumulated and maternal rubella infection has come to be recognized as one of the major causes of congenital defects. Considerable research was carried out to find means of preventing maternal rubella but was hampered by difficulties in isolating the virus, which was not accomplished until 1962.[1] On isolation of the virus,efforts turned toward the development of a vaccine and an attenuated live virus vaccine was developed in 1965[2] and licensed and approved for use in July 1969.

Before going into the use of the vaccine and its effects, I think we should briefly review the teratogenicity of the rubella virus. Approximately nine days after infection, viremia occurs during which the virus can infect and cross the placenta to infect the fetus. Having infected the fetus, the type of defect produced appears to be dependent on the developmental stage of the fetus. The risk of congenital deformity is related to the stage of pregnancy at the time of infection. Table 1, showing data from the Rubella Birth Defect Evaluation Project of Dr. Cooper at New York University,[3] shows the clinical status of 370 children born to women suspected of having rubella during pregnancy. As the population was selected retrospectively, it is likely that the rates of abnormalities are higher than they would be if the population had been identified prospectively and, in fact, the Collaborative Perinatal Research Study[4] found a 16.7% rate of congenital rubella following first trimester maternal rubella. Whichever rate is true, it is clear that there is an extremely high rate of abnormality in infants born to women infected during the first

129

TABLE 1

Clinical Status of 370 Children and Time of Maternal Rubella

Maternal Rubella	Number Abnormal/Total	Percent Abnormal
First Month	56/60	93.3
Second Month	101/106	95.3
Third Month	64/82	78.0
Fourth Month	22/43	51.2
> Fourth Month	1/16	6.2
No Clinical Rubella	42/44	95.5
Insufficient Information	14/19	73.7

Source: Cooper, *et al.*, 1969

two months of pregnancy and that this rate falls off in later stages of pregnancy. A variety of congenital defects can be produced by the virus and Table 2, again from Dr. Cooper's study,[3] shows the frequency of specific defects in his population. Deafness was the most common abnormality seen, followed by heart disease, psychomotor retardation, and cataracts. Multiple defects were common, and only about one quarter of the children had only a single defect. Of the cardiovascular defects, the most common were patent ductus arteriosis, right pulmonary artery stenosis, left pulmonary artery stenosis, in descending order of frequency. Of the 61 deaths during the first four years of life, most occurred during the first year of life "...and were associated with congestive heart failure, sepsis and general debility".[3]

Many infants affected *in utero* with rubella virus will excrete the virus after birth and virus excretion for as long as 18 months after birth has been documented. Thus these infants are potential sources of infection for other children, pregnant women and hospital personnel.

Although most of the defects mentioned above are fairly severe, a 25 year follow-up study of 50 patients with congenital rubella[5] revealed surprising adjustment of most patients even though 48 were deaf, 26 had rubella cataracts or chorioretinopathy and 11 had congenital cardiovascular defects. In spite of this, all but four were employed at the time of follow-up. This sample is admittedly biased since it included only persons who had survived the first years of life. Nonetheless, it appears that those born with congenital rubella defects who make it through the first few years of life have a reasonable opportunity for adaptation to society.

Public and scientific concern was directed even more strongly toward the prevention of congenital rubella infection by the massive epidemic of rubella which occurred in the United States in 1964 and in which it is estimated that there were 20,000 children born alive with rubella defects and an additional 12,000 abortions or stillbirths resulting from maternal infection.[6] It has been postulated that this large number of affected infants resulted from some change in the teratogenicity of the rubella virus but this opinion does not seem to be widely held.[7,8]

In 1965, Meyer and Parkman selected a virus which had been passed in African green monkey kidney culture as being satisfactory for clinical evaluation.[2] Between that time and the licensure of the vaccine in 1969, several things were learned about the vaccine virus which had considerable bearing on the ultimate use of the vaccine and on the controversy regarding the approach being taken in this country. These factors included the fact that the vaccine virus produces viremia and is capable of infecting the placenta and fetus, questions regarding the duration of immunity and the degree of immunity as related to reinfection, and side effects of the vaccine itself. Let us consider

TABLE 2

Frequency of Defects Among 376 Children Born Following Maternal Rubella

Defect	Number	Percent
None	70	18.6
Deafness	252	67.0
Heart Disease	182	48.4
Psychomotor Retardation	170	45.2
Retinopathy	147	39.1
Cataract (s)	108	28.7
Purpura	85	22.6
Glaucoma	12	3.2
Deaths	61	16.2

Source: Cooper, *et al.*, 1969

these factors briefly:

1. It is well known that the vaccine virus can produce viremia and that the vaccine virus is capable of infecting the placenta. What is not known is the likelihood of production of congenital defect in infants born to mothers receiving vaccine during pregnancy. Table 3 is a composite of the national experience with women vaccinated immediately preceding or during pregnancy. The data were obtained by the Center for Disease Control.[9] Of 215 women known to have received rubella vaccine immediately preceding or during pregnancy, 44% carried their pregnancies to term and delivered normal term infants with the exception of one child who had cystic fibrosis. This would suggest that the teratogenicity of the vaccine virus is of lesser magnitude than that of the wild virus. However, it must be noted that only 11 women known to be susceptible to rubella at the time of immunization carried their infants to term. One half of the women underwent therapeutic abortion because of the fear of vaccine-induced congenital deformity. Viral studies were performed on products of conception in a significant proportion of these. Vaccine-like virus was recovered from four products of conception of the susceptible women, in one instance from the fetal eye, in two from the placenta and in one from decidual tissue. Of the women of unknown immune status, vaccine-like virus was recovered from three products of conception: once from fetal eye and placenta, once from fetal kidney and placenta and once from placenta alone. This clearly demonstrates the ability of the virus to infect placental and fetal tissues.

2. Questions have also arisen regarding the duration and degree of immunity conferred by vaccination. Antibody levels following vaccination are generally not as high as those following natural illness and the vaccine has been available for a short enough time that it is difficult to know whether immunity will be lifelong. It should be pointed out that in these respects rubella vaccine is much like measles vaccine at the time of its introduction. However, the concern over the possibility of sub-clinical reinfection with rubella virus is greater than for measles virus because of the possibility of fetal infection. It has been shown that immunized individuals can be reinfected with rubella virus and that a boost in antibody levels will result, suggesting true infection. Vaccine has been recovered from the pharynx of these reinfected individuals but viremia has not been demonstrated.[10] Consequently, we are not at this point in a position to confirm or deny the possibility of fetal infection in reinfected immunized individuals.

3. The last vaccine-related factor I want to mention is that of side effects from the vaccine, specifically arthralgia following vaccination. Arthralgia and frank arthritis have been reported in vaccinees since the first field trials of rubella vaccine. It has since become apparent that the incidence of these joint

133

TABLE 3

Outcome of Pregnancy in 215 Women Receiving Rubella Vaccine Immediately
Preceding or During Pregnancy

U. S. Totals Through June 1972

Immune Status	Total	Therapeutic Abortion	Spontaneous Abortion	Term Delivery
Susceptible	24	10	3	11
Immune	7	0	0	7
Unknown	184	97	9	78
Total	215	107	12	96[*]

[*]All term births were normal except for one infant with cystic fibrosis.

Source: CDC

reactions depends to a certain extent on the type of vaccine used, with the dog kidney preparation causing more joint reactions than the more widely used duck embryo or rabbit kidney preparations.[10-12] It is also apparent that joint reactions are more frequent in older vaccinees, with rates as high as 25 to 30% in adult females in some studies.[10]

Taking into account all of these factors related to the vaccine and those relating to the epidemiology of the disease, two schools of thought developed regarding the best use of rubella vaccine to prevent congenital rubella infection. The first school favored the direct approach of immunizing individuals at risk of contracting infection while pregnant. Thus, this group would favor the immunization of adolescent and adult females. The other school of thought favored the vaccination of young children since they are the primary transmitters of the disease.

With regard to the direct approach, it obviously would protect those who are at immediate risk. However, about 85% of adult females in the United States are immune to rubella and in no need of immunization. Consequently, some means of determining their susceptibility is necessary. Individual recall of having had rubella is not particularly accurate. Lerman[13] has shown that 8% of women with a history of rubella were susceptible by antibody testing and that 45% of those without a history of rubella were susceptible. The other side of this is that 55% of those who denied a history of rubella were shown to be immune. Immune status can only be determined accurately by performance of a rubella antibody test and this test is not presently available everywhere in the United States. Additionally, because of the possible teratogenicity of the vaccine virus it is essential that vaccinees not be pregnant at the time of vaccination and that they do not become pregnant within the six weeks to two months following vaccination. This poses an additional problem in patient management, and one that is well demonstrated by the figures in Table 3, showing that there have been at least 215 pregnant or soon-to-become pregnant women vaccinated and that only 11% of them were known to be susceptible and in need of immunization.

Additionally, it should be pointed out that this approach would have little effect on the overall persistence of rubella virus in the country.

Regarding the indirect approach, it is clear that the individuals with highest incidence of rubella were young children, specifically those in the 5 to 9 year age group who frequently brought the infection home from school to the rest of the family.[14] Vaccination of this group should reduce the general prevalence of rubella virus and curtail transmission of the virus to pregnant women. Against this approach is the fact that we are not sure that immunity would last through the individual's period of risk in a girl immunized as a young child and that a false sense of security might be built up by vaccinating

135

transmission can occur in a setting with high levels of immunity.[15-18]   This has been countered by evidence showing that epidemics of rubella can be curtailed by administration of rubella vaccine.[19-20]

After balancing all these factors the American Academy of Pediatrics and the Public Health Service Advisory Committee on Immunization Practice recommended the adoption of the indirect approach, with vaccination recommended for all children between the age of 1 and puberty. Here in New York State, the Legislature passed a law requiring rubella immunization as a condition for school entry effective September 1970. Great Britain and some other countries have adopted the direct approach and there remains in this country considerable sentiment in favor of the direct approach.

Following the licensure of the vaccine and the policy recommendations, a nationwide program, heavily financed with federal funds, was undertaken to immunize our children. By July 1, 1972, only three years after licensure of the vaccine, over 28 million doses of rubella vaccine had been administered in public programs and it was estimated that 78.5% of all 5 to 9 year olds in the nation and 54.6% of all 1 to 4 year olds had been immunized.[21] Figure 1 shows the correlation between national monthly incidence of rubella and cumulative usage of rubella vaccine from 1966 through September 1972. There is clearly a declining incidence of rubella as reported to health departments which is temporarily associated with the rising number of children vaccinated. Here in New York State, we have had a more or less similar experience. Figure 2 shows, for New York State exclusive of New York City, monthly incidence of rubella since January 1966 and cumulative number of children vaccinated against rubella in public programs. Once again a decline can be seen in the incidence of rubella concomitant with the increasing utilization of vaccine.

Whether or not this decline is a result of our rubella vaccination program can obviously not be answered with certainty although I believe there are data that support this view. For each of the six years 1964 through 1969 the 5 to 9 year age group had the highest incidence rate of rubella in New York. In 1970 and 1971 this age group, which is the age group best immunized, dropped to third and fourth place respectively and first place was taken over by infants under the age of 1, a group which is not being vaccinated.

These data may indicate that rubella in general is becoming less common as a result of the immunization program but what is happening to the incidence of congenital rubella syndrome? This obviously is the best indicator of the success of our approach. Table 4 shows the number of cases of congenital rubella syndrome reported in the United States from 1966 through September 1972 (prior to 1966 it was not reportable).[22] The peak reported incidence was reached in 1970 and it has been declining since then. This might be taken as an indication that our approach is working and I wish I could say that it

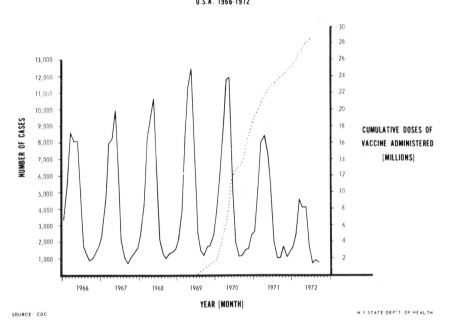

RUBELLA INCIDENCE AND CUMULATIVE RUBELLA VACCINE USE

U.S.A. 1966-1972

SOURCE: CDC

N.Y.STATE DEP'T. OF HEALTH

Figure 1

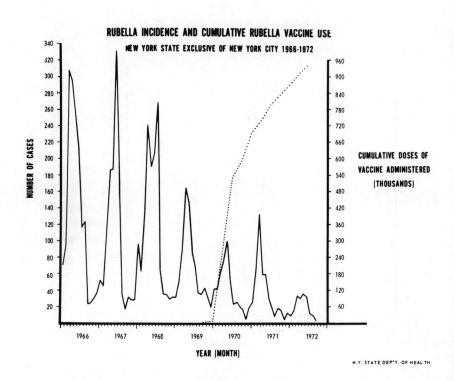

Figure 2

TABLE 4

Reported Congenital Rubella Syndrome – U. S. A.

1966 – 1972

Year	Number
1966	11
1967	10
1968	14
1969	31
1970	77
1971	68
1972	25[*]

*Through September

Source: CDC

was such an indication. Unfortunately, we have no accurate way of knowing whether this apparent decline in incidence is real or not. It is obvious that our reporting system for congenital rubella syndrome is poor and it is quite likely that the peak incidence demonstrated in 1970 resulted from peak enthusiasm regarding reporting and that reporting has dropped as a result of waning enthusiasm since then. Although reporting of congenital rubella syndrome is mandatory in virtually every state in the nation (although not yet in New York for unknown reasons), it is clear that merely passing such a requirement does not get results. Surveillance of congenital rubella syndrome involves active solicitation of reports from pediatricians and from centers likely to be seeing children who have defects due to rubella such as schools for the deaf, etc., and such a system is not yet operative in most parts of the country.

I am thus in the unhappy position of having to conclude by saying that our indirect approach to the prevention of congenital rubella syndrome must presently be evaluated by indirect means, that is, by monitoring the incidence of clinical rubella infection.

REFERENCES

1. J.A. Forbes, *Amer. J. Dis. Child. 118*, 5, 1969.

2. H.M. Meyer, P.D. Parkman and T.E. Hobbins *et al.*, *Amer. J. Dis. Child. 118*, 155, 1969.

3. L.Z. Cooper, P.R. Ziring and A.B. Ockerse *et al.*, *Amer. J. Dis. Child. 118*, 18, 1969.

4. J.L. Sever, J.B. Hardy and K.B. Nelson *et al.*, *Amer. J. Dis. Child. 118*, 123, 1969.

5. M.A. Menser, L. Dods and J.D. Harley, *Lancet* 1347, 1967.

6. S. Shavell, National Communicable Disease Center Rubella Surveillance, *1*, 11, 1969.

7. L.R. White, J.L. Sever and F.P. Alepa, *Pediatrics 74*, 198, 1969.

8. M. Siegel, H.T. Fuerst and V.F. Guinee, *Amer. J. Dis. Child. 121*, 469, 1971.

9. Center for Disease Control, personal communications, 1972.

10. H.M. Meyer and P.D. Parkman, *J.A.M.A. 215*, 613, 1971.

11. S.M. Austin, R. Altman and E.K. Barnes *et al., Amer J. Epid. 95,* 53, 1972.

12. E.K. Barnes, R. Altman and S.M. Austin *et al., Amer. J. Epid. 95,* 59, 1972.

13. S.J. Lerman, L.M. Lerman and G.A. Nankervis *et al., Annals Int. Med. 74,* 97, 1971.

14. New York State Department of Health. Unpublished data.

15. T.W. Chang, S. DesRosiers and L. Weinstein, *New. Engl. J. Med. 283,* 246, 1970.

16. W.J. Davis, H.E. Larson and J.P. Simsarian *et al., J.A.M.A. 215,* 600, 1971.

17. D.E. Lehane, N.R. Newberg and W. E. Beam, *J.A.M.A. 213,* 2236, 1970.

18. D.M. Horstmann, H. Liebhaber and G.L. LeBouvier *et al., New Engl. J. Med. 283,* 778, 1970.

19. R.G. Judelsohn, Termination of a rubella outbreak in Bermuda by vaccination. Presented at Annual Convention of the American Public Health Association, 1971.

20. T. Furukawa, T. Miyata and K. Kondo *et al., J.A.M.A. 213,* 987, 1970.

21. Center for Disease Control, Rubella, Measles, Polio Immunization Status Report 2 (No.12), 1972.

22. Center for Disease Control, Morbidity and Mortality Weekly Reports Annual Summaries, 1966–1971 (Nos. 1–39), 1972.

DISCUSSION

DR. LILIENFELD: Dr. Flynt, you spoke of the observed changes in the frequency of limb reduction deformities as being significant. As I recall, you reported a birth population base of 30,000 in Atlanta. What statistical procedures are yielding significance for the relatively small change which you observed?

DR. FLYNT: The results are based on the long term trends. The procedure statistically predicts what one would have expected for the time period and the observed number of births.

DR. NEEL: Dr. Flynt, have you asked whether there is heterogeneity in your series? When you are dealing with small numbers in examining data on a monthly basis, a change from three cases in a month to five cases in a month might be statistically significant. However, I wonder if that small change should be considered significant in the teratogenic sense?

DR. FLYNT: The statistical system should not be interpreted literally. It is a sentinal device which ensures that each defect is looked at in the same way during each time period. One of the overriding questions is, when does one become concerned about an observed increase? We became a little more concerned because there had been reports of increases in reduction deformities from other countries.

DR. NEEL: I'm afraid that unless one becomes concerned on the basis of sound statistical principles, we're apt to have "much ado about nothing", rather frequently.

GABRIEL STICKLES (National Foundation March of Dimes, White Plains, New York): I'm afraid if we delay our concern until we can prove something, we may delay until it is too late.

ROSALIE GREEN: Dr. Flynt, have you asked whether any of these women were using sex hormones or female hormones or birth prevention before their pregnancy? The effect of possible teratogenesis during the pregnancy isn't the entire issue and matters such as hormones should be explored.

DR. FLYNT: Yes, we have asked about the use of sex hormones and the oral contraceptives. In special follow-up studies such as this one, we

143

question the mother about any area which we feel is pertinent. However, we always have to be careful about data which is based upon recall or mothers' memory.

DR. HOOK: In defense of the system which Dr. Flynt has described, it is not surprising that there will be fluctuations in the background causes of birth defects. We may, in fact, be seeing, or it may be difficult to tell, what is an increase in incidence to some, presumably introduced, teratogen rather than some fluctuation in background causes. But despite that difficulty, it is still important that all apparent increases in frequency be investigated as thoroughly as possible. Clearly, the type of investigation must be related to the energies and to the talents of those available. So, I think the question of at what level do you investigate an increase is perhaps not quite as important as that the increase be investigated. If a particular environmental cause is not found, there should not be pessimism about the failure to turn one up. This remains purely a personal view of this. Again, the question of the exact statistical significance is less important than the question of getting at the environmental causes. Perhaps that was addressed more to Dr. Neel than to Dr. Flynt.

DR. LILIENFELD: I would like to underline that. It seems to me that a monitoring system should be sensitive to pick up departures from the normal. From that viewpoint, it would seem to me that it is quite justifiable to say that this is an increase which should set up the follow-up investigative system. The question comes up, though, once you've recognized it and you've followed up, you must make a definite inference as to whether a real increase has occurred. Follow-up is needed in order to make that determination.

DR. NEEL: Dr. Hook, I'd like to think I'm as worried about monitoring as anybody else. But let me propose this situation: if your system is too sensitive, and you have 30 different indicators, one or two of them would be expected to sound the alarm each month purely on the basis of chance. So it seems to me that we have to hit a proper level here. I'm not sure we saw the proper levels at this point, largely because the statistical approach has not been presented. If you do not make the system sensitive enough, you're certainly going to miss something. We have to work out the proper middle course.

DR. NANCE: I'd like to point out one nationwide source of data on the incidence of deafness which might be worth looking at in monitoring for rubella deafness. This is the annual survey of hearing impaired children and youths. This survey is conducted by a college in Washington. They collect data on some 25,000 deaf children from 400 reporting sources around the country. When you examine the incidence of deafness by year of birth in this population sample, you can clearly see the epidemic nature of the affliction, which presumably is attributable to rubella.

DR. HINMAN: The only problem with that type of data is that it is difficult to determine deafness at an early age — in infancy, for example. Then one is faced with the problem of retrospective data. Our problem is that we want to know what effect the immunization program is having presently. Several years from now, I think we should be able to get a complete picture by monitoring such retrospective data. But I'm afraid that at the present time they're not much help to us.

STEVEN PAUKER: Is the rubella vaccine virus transmissible to people in the same way as the polio virus?

DR. HINMAN: No, there have been fairly extensive studies of susceptible populations in contact with immunized individuals, and to my knowledge there have been only two instances in which apparent spread of the vaccine virus has been demonstrated from a vaccinated individual to a susceptible individual who was in close contact. One very nice study in Hawaii with young adults used married couples who were both sero-negative and vaccinated one partner of each of the couples and followed them fairly closely. One assumes that they were undergoing quite close contact yet there was no instance of sero-conversion in that group.

DR. STICKLES: Can you, or anyone else from the New York State Department of Health, explain why New York State ranks 50th among the states in the proportion of children vaccinated against rubella?

DR. HINMAN: Yes, I think it has to do with how one generates the data. We are in the process of conducting a statewide immunization survey which will give us a valid indication of the proportion of children in New York state who are vaccinated against rubella. The problem with the nationally published figures is that they list only vaccinations given in public clinics. They do not take into account vaccinations given in the private sector. In a county such as Nassau County in New York, which has the lowest proportion of children vaccinated in public clinics, the most likely answer is that Nassau County is a fairly prosperous county and a high proportion of children in this area are receiving their care from private physicians. They are probably receiving their immunizations in the same way. That is one of the reasons we're anxiously awaiting the results of our statewide immunization survey. I think it will show that we are not in 50th place.

DR. LILIENFELD: Dr. Hinman, was the number of couples included in the study which you mentioned sufficient to eliminate the possibility of transmissibility?

DR. HINMAN: No, it was not. However, a number of other studies have been reported and they indicate that the likelihood of transmission is extremely small.

SECTION IV

STILBESTROL EXPOSURE IN UTERO: LONG TERM EFFECT*

P. Greenwald
P. C. Nasca

In New York State, nine teenage girls are known to have developed vaginal or cervical cancer after their mothers took stilbestrol or another synthetic estrogen during pregnancy. Six of these girls have died of advanced disease. This paper will review the study of these nine patients, with particular reference to the dosage level and latency. Data on stilbestrol in relation to animal and other human tumors will also be presented. Five of these patients have previously been reported.[1]

REPORTS OF VAGINAL CANCER

Physicians, hospitals and laboratories throughout New York State are required by State law to report all patients with cancer to a registry maintained by the Health Department. New York City was recently added to this reporting system. The registry, supplemented by a letter from State Health Commissioner, Dr. Hollis S. Ingraham, requesting reports from each of the 37,500 practicing physicians in the State, served as the initial source of information on the nine patients. We believe that all diagnosed vaginal tumors in women under 30 years old were reported for further study.

The nine patients were studied in detail for a history of drug use by their mothers during pregnancy. Stilbestrol was definitely given to the mothers of seven patients. Confirmation of synthetic estrogen use by the mother of each patient was obtained from careful review of both the hospital and attending physician's obstetrical records in addition to interviews with these mothers. Obstetricians used the therapy to prevent threatened abortion. The mother of the eighth patient told us herself that she had received therapy during pregnancy in order to avoid "a miscarriage like the last time". Destruction of records, however, prevented definite ascertainment of whether stilbestrol was used. The ninth patient took another non-steroidal synthetic estrogen,

*Supported in part by a grant (CA 12707-01) from the National Cancer Institute.

used. The ninth patient took another non-steroidal synthetic estrogen, dienestrol, which is very similar to stilbestrol.

A control group was developed by matching vaginal cancer patients with female infants born at the same hospital at about the same time to mothers of the same five-year age group and with the same number of previous children. Matching was done with the aid of birth certificates on file in the Health Department. None of the mothers of control subjects received stilbestrol therapy during pregnancy. At time of diagnosis, the patients ranged in age from 15 to 19 years. Place of birth varied widely with four patients being born in upstate New York, four in New York City and one in Pennsylvania.

Histologically, all tumors resembled those described by Herbst and his colleagues in their original reports[2,3] containing the characteristic clear cells and "hobnail" cells.

All patients were single and had no children. Their menstrual periods one year before the first symptoms were described as normal, and none had hormone or contraceptive therapy before the onset of the first symptom.

Drs. Herbst, Poskanzer, Scully and Ulfelder of the Vincent Memorial and Massachusetts General Hospitals, Boston, have been collecting reports of vaginal and cervical adenocarcinoma from throughout the country, including those reported here. At the present time, over eighty patients have been reported. The range of age at diagnosis is 8 to 24 years, and several patients had borne children prior to diagnosis.

DOSE AND LATENCY

Synthetic estrogen therapy was begun during the first trimester for the mothers of all nine patients. The mean duration of therapy was five months with a range of 2½ to 9 months.

Approximate cumulative dosages of synthetic estrogens taken during pregnancy for the nine mothers of vaginal cancer patients and 21 mothers of patients whose children did not develop cancer are shown in Table 1. Among mothers of patients, the mean total dose was 2316 mg and the range 450 to 4875. The dosage taken by mothers of cancer patients was compared to mothers of the nine non-ill daughters on whom data are available. (Mothers of sons were excluded from the significance test on the means because the sons would have no possibility of developing the tumors of concern.) There is no significant difference in the mean dosages of the two groups of mothers. However, very few women in either group received small dosages, and thus it would not be possible to determine a dose-response gradient from these data. Animal studies[4] have shown that the carcinogenic effect is retained at low levels of administration.

TABLE 1

Amount of Synthetic Estrogen Taken During Pregnancy by Mothers of Vaginal Cancer Children and Non-ill Children, New York State, 1950–1972

		Non-ill Children Maternal Synthetic Estrogen				Vaginal Cancer Children Maternal Synthetic Estrogen		
No.	Sex of Child	Average daily Dose (mg)	Number of Days	Total Dose (mg)	No.	Average daily Dose (mg)	Number of Days	Total Dose (mg)
1.	Male	4	120	480	1.	5	90	450
2.	Male	5	120	600	2.	7	90	630
3.	Female	30	30	900	3.	8	180	1440
4.	Male	8	120	960	4.	25	90	2250
5.	Male	10	120	1200	5.	11	270	2970
6.	Female	12	120	1440	6.	15	240	3600
7.	Male	10	150	1500	7.	65	75	4875
8.	Male	10	150	1500	8.	Unknown	180	—
9.	Female	12	180	2160	9.	Unknown	180	—
10.	Male	15	150	2250				
11.	Male	18	150	2700				
12.	Female	16	180	2880				
13.	Female	16	180	2880				
14.	Male	16	180	2880				
15.	Female	19	180	3420				
16.	Male	20	180	3600				
17.	Female	21	180	3780				
18.	Male	40	150	6000				
19.	Female	50	120	6000				
20.	Female	50	120	6000				
21.	Male	50	150	7500				
	Mothers of Female Children Only (N=9)							
Mean		25	143	3273 mg		(N=7) 19	(N=9) 155	(N=7) 2316 mg
S. D.		15	51	1792 mg		21	72	1619 mg

t tests - p >.05 for differences between means.

151

Month of gestation at start of synthetic estrogen therapy and duration of therapy are shown in Table 2. It can be seen that for all cases, therapy was begun during the first trimester, while for one-third of the controls (female children only) it was begun later. There was no significant difference in duration of therapy.

Date of birth for cases and controls (Table 3) shows that all patients were born during the period 1951 through 1955, the time of peak clinical use of stilbestrol to prevent miscarriages. There were no significant differences in month of birth.

The New York State patients were 15 to 19 years old at time of diagnosis. As noted above, the range at age of diagnosis for all reported cases in the United States is 8 to 24 years, although most were in their late teens. Table 4 shows how this latent period compares with the latent periods of some other carcinogens in man. While there are clearly differences in age at exposure, type of carcinogen and mechanism of exposure, this comparison offers no reason for thinking that we should not expect some patients with longer latency periods to be diagnosed as the interval since the peak years of stilbestrol exposure grows longer.

OTHER TUMOR TYPES

Animal studies have shown that stilbestrol can be made to induce a variety of tumor types in several species. The tumors are primarily of endocrine-related or urinary organs.[4,5]

In order to investigate the possibility that tumors of organs other than the vagina might also be associated with maternal stilbestrol use, prenatal drug use histories were obtained on mothers of all female patients in upstate New York born after 1947 and reported with cancers of the breast, uterine cervix (adenocarcinoma only), uterine corpus, fallopian tube, vagina (sarcoma botryoides), and urethra, and all males born after 1947 and reported with cancer of the breast, prostate, penis, epididymis, spermatic cord and urethra.[6] A number of patients with cancers of the adrenal, pituitary, ovary, testis, bladder and kidney were also studied. The rationale for the selection of sites favored glands which produce sex hormones or are target organs for these hormones, are male homologues of the female vagina and uterus, develop embryologically from the urogenital ridge, or are sites to which rare tumors of these organs might have been misclassified during registration.

Results of these histories and animal tumor responses to stilbestrol are shown on Tables 5A, 5B and 5C. The animal data are taken from published studies[4,5] and no attempt was made to check the validity of the observations. Stilbestrol was taken during pregnancy by the mother of only one patient,

TABLE 2

Month of Gestation Started and Length of Stilbestrol Therapy

Month of Gestation Therapy Started	Total	Length of Therapy (Months)								
		1	2	3	4	5	6	7	8	9
Cases (Female Children Only)										
Total	9	—	1	3	—	—	3	—	1	1
1	3	—	—	1	—	—	—	—	1	1
2	0	—	—	—	—	—	—	—	—	—
3	6	—	1	2	—	—	3	—	—	—
4	0	—	—	—	—	—	—	—	—	—
5	0	—	—	—	—	—	—	—	—	—
Controls (Male and Female Children)										
Total	21	1	—	—	7	6	7	—	—	—
1	0	—	—	—	—	—	—	—	—	—
2	0	—	—	—	—	—	—	—	—	—
3	16	1	—	—	3	5	7	—	—	—
4	3	—	—	—	2	1	—	—	—	—
5	2	—	—	—	2	—	—	—	—	—
Controls (Female Children Only)										
Total	9	1	—	—	3	—	5	—	—	—
1	0	—	—	—	—	—	—	—	—	—
2	0	—	—	—	—	—	—	—	—	—
3	6	1	—	—	—	—	5	—	—	—
4	2	—	—	—	2	—	—	—	—	—
5	1	—	—	—	1	—	—	—	—	—

TABLE 3
Date of Birth of Children of Mothers Using Stilbestrol

Year	Total	Jan.	Feb.	Mar.	Apr.	May	June	July	Aug.	Sept.	Oct.	Nov.	Dec.	N.S.
Cases (Female Only)														
Total	9	–	2	–	3	–	–	–	1	1	1	–	–	1
1951	1	–	1	–	–	–	–	–	–	–	–	–	–	–
1952	5	–	1	–	2	–	–	–	–	1	1	–	–	–
1953	2	–	–	–	1	–	–	–	1	–	–	–	–	–
1954	0	–	–	–	–	–	–	–	–	–	–	–	–	–
1955	1	–	–	–	–	–	–	–	–	–	–	–	–	1
Controls (Males and Females)														
Total	21	2	1	–	2	4	1	2	1	1	4	1	2	–
1949	1	–	–	–	–	–	–	–	–	–	–	–	–	–
1950	3	1	–	–	1	–	–	–	–	1	–	1	–	–
1951	2	1	–	–	1	–	–	–	–	–	1	–	1	–
1952	3	1	–	–	–	1	–	–	–	–	1	–	–	–
1953	3	–	–	–	–	–	–	–	–	–	2	–	–	–
1954	2	–	–	–	1	2	1	–	–	–	–	–	1	–
1955	3	–	–	–	–	–	–	–	–	–	–	–	–	–
1956	0	–	–	–	–	–	–	–	–	–	–	–	–	–
1957	0	–	–	–	–	–	–	–	–	–	–	–	–	–
1958	0	–	–	–	–	–	–	–	–	–	–	–	–	–
1959	0	–	–	–	–	–	–	–	–	–	–	–	–	–
1960	1	–	–	–	–	–	–	–	–	–	–	–	–	–
1961	0	–	–	–	–	–	–	–	1	–	–	–	–	–
1962	1	–	–	–	–	–	–	–	–	–	–	–	–	–
Controls (Females Only)														
Total	9	1	1	2	2	–	–	1	1	1	1	1	1	–
1949	2	1	–	–	2	–	–	–	–	–	–	–	–	–
1950	1	1	–	–	–	–	–	–	–	–	–	1	–	–
1951	1	–	–	–	–	–	–	1	–	–	–	–	1	–
1952	0	–	–	–	–	–	–	–	–	–	–	–	–	–
1953	1	–	–	–	–	–	–	–	–	–	–	–	–	–
1954	1	–	–	–	1	–	–	–	–	–	–	–	–	–
1955	0	–	–	–	–	–	–	–	–	–	–	–	–	–
1956	1	–	–	–	–	–	–	–	–	–	1	–	–	–
1957	0	–	–	–	–	–	–	–	–	–	–	–	–	–
1958	1	–	1	–	–	–	–	–	–	–	–	–	–	–
1959	0	–	–	–	–	–	–	–	–	–	–	–	–	–
1960	0	–	–	–	–	–	–	–	–	–	–	–	–	–
1961	0	–	–	–	–	–	–	–	–	–	–	–	–	–
1962	1	–	–	–	–	–	–	–	1	–	–	–	–	–

154

TABLE 4

Latent Periods of Selected Cancers[a]

Organ and Agent	Average Latent Period Years	Range of Latent Period Years
Vagina and Cervix		
Stilbestrol	17	8—24
Skin		
Arsenic:		
Medicinal	18	3—40
Occupational	25	4—46
Tar	20—24	1—50
Creosote oil	25	15—40
Mineral oil	50—54	4—75
Crude paraffin oil	15—18	3—35
Solar radiation	20—30	15—40
X-radiation	7	1—12
Lung		
Asbestos	18	15—21
Chromates	15	5—47
Nickel	22	6—30
Tar fumes	16	9—23
Ionizing radiation	25—35	7—50
Bladder		
Aromatic amines	11—15	2—40

[a]Data on cancers related to occupational exposure are taken from W.C. Hueper and W.D. Conway, *in* Chemical Carcinogenesis and Cancers, 1964. Courtesy of Charles C. Thomas, Publisher, Springfield, Illinois.

Comparison of Animal Tumor Response to Stilbestrol and History of Maternal Estrogen Therapy in
Patients Born After 1947 and Reported to the New York State Cancer Registry With Tumors of the Same Sites

Species	Sex	Tumor Type	Sex	Number Studied	Tumor Type	Maternal Stilbestrol History
	ANIMAL[a]				HUMAN	
BREAST TUMORS						
Mouse	M	Adenocarcinoma	M	0[c]		
		Adenoacanthoma	F	3[d]	Adenocarcinoma	Negative
	F	Adenocarcinoma				
		Adenoacanthoma				
		Carcinosarcoma				
		Benign tumor				
Rat	F	Carcinoma				
		Benign tumor				
PITUITARY TUMORS						
Mouse	M	Adenoma	M	2	Craniopharyngioma	Negative
	F	Chromophobe adenoma	F	1	Craniopharyngioma	Negative
		Adenoma		1	Chromophobe carcinoma	Negative
Rat	M	Adenoma				
	F	Adenoma				
Hamster	M	Pituitary tumors				
		Chromophobe adenoma				
ADRENAL TUMORS						
Mouse	M	Cortical carcinoma	M	3	Neuroblastoma	Negative
	F	Pheochromocytoma		1	Adenocarcinoma	Negative
Rat	F	Carcinoma	F	3	Adenocarcinoma	Negative
OVARIAN TUMORS						
Rat	F	Fibrosarcoma	F	2	Mesonephroma	Negative
TESTICULAR TUMORS						
Mouse	M	Testicular tumor	M	2	Clear cell adenocarcinoma	Negative
Hamster	M	Adenoma				
UTERINE TUMORS						
Mouse	F	Utero-cervical carcinoma	F	1[d]	Adenocarcinoma (Cervix and Vagina)	Positive
	F	Fibrosarcoma				
Rabbit	F	Adenocarcinoma		4[d]	Sarcoma (Corpus)	Negative
		Luteoma		2[d]	Adenoacanthoma	Negative
VAGINAL AND VULVAL TUMORS						
Mouse	F	Cervico-vaginal epidermoid carcinoma	F	4[d]	Sarcoma Botryoides	Negative
		Vulval epidermoid carcinoma				
Rat	F	Papilloma				
KIDNEY TUMORS						
Mouse	M	Carcinoma	M	2	Clear cell adenocarcinoma	Negative
Hamster	M	Carcinoma				
		Papillary cystadenoma	F	1	Clear cell adenocarcinoma	Negative
	F	Malignant tumor				
BLADDER TUMORS						
Rat[b]	M		M	6	Transitional cell	Negative
				1	Sarcoma Botryoides	Negative
	F			1	Rhabdomyosarcoma	Negative
			F	4	Transitional cell	Negative
				1	Rhabdomyosarcoma	Negative

[a]Source: Reference 4
[b]Source: Reference 5
[c]No reported cases
[d]All reported cases born after 1947

TABLE 5B

History of Maternal Estrogen Therapy in Patients Born After 1947 and Reported to the New York State Cancer Registry With Tumors of Sites Not Noted in Table 5A

Site	Sex	Number Studied	Tumor Type	Maternal Stilbestrol History
Prostate	M	10 [a]	Sarcoma	Negative
Epididymis	M	1 [d]	Sarcoma	Negative
Spermatic Cord	M	2 [d]	Rhabdomyosarcoma	Negative
Urethra	M	1 [d]	Transitional cell carcinoma	Negative
Retroperitoneal	F	1	Meso-metanephroma	Negative

[a]All reported cases born after 1947.

157

TABLE 5C

Other Stilbestrol-induced Animal Tumors Reported in the Literature[a]

Site	Animal	Sex	Pathology
Subcutaneous	Mouse	M	Reticulum Cell Sarcoma
			Fibrosarcoma
		F	Fibrosarcoma
Bone	Mouse	F	Osteogenic Sarcoma
Blood vessels	Mouse	M	Hemangioendotheliomas
		F	Hemangioendotheliomas
Blood	Rat	F	Leukemia
Liver	Mouse	M	Hepatoma
		F	Hepatoma
			Reticulum Cell Sarcoma
Brain	Mouse	F	Glioblastoma Multiforme
Lung	Mouse	M	Pulmonary tumors
		F	Pulmonary tumors

[a]Source: Reference 4

an 18-year old girl with adenocarcinoma involving both the cervix and vagina. The exact site of primary lesion could not be determined. These data plus analysis of site, age and sex-specific time trends of tumor registry data show no indication thus far that maternal use of stilbestrol contributes to the development of tumors other than those of the lower female genital tract.

DISCUSSION

In this report, nine teenage girls are described whose mothers received synthetic estrogens during pregnancy. Denominator data on how many New York State women received these hormones during pregnancy are necessary to calculate risk and are not available. A rather small risk, however, is suggested by evidence of widespread use of stilbestrol in the early 1950's as derived from interviews with obstetricians and supported by the broad geographical area of birth of the patients. In addition, a review of delivery records of forty diabetic mothers living in the Syracuse area who delivered between 1950 and 1955 revealed that 14 had been given stilbestrol. Further evidence to provide hope that the risk may be low comes in recent reports from the Mayo Clinic.[7] These investigators found that 1,340 residents of Rochester, Minnesota received estrogens during pregnancy in the years 1946 through 1954, but none of the daughters of these pregnancies are known to have developed vaginal or cervical adenocarcinoma.

The Mayo Clinic report describes three patients with cervical adenocarcinoma whose mothers took synthetic estrogens. It is clear from this study, the work of Herbst and his colleagues and our own data, that the same maternal drug association exists for clear-cell adenocarcinoma of the cervix as exists for vaginal cancer.

Indeed, women taking stilbestrol over a long period possibly are themselves at increased risk for endometrial cancer. Cutler et al[8] reported five patients, including three from the literature, with endometrial carcinoma developing after prolonged stilbestrol treatment for gonadal dysgenesis. Three of the tumors were of an unusual mixed or adenosquamous type. Endometrial cancer has also been reported after prolonged estrogen therapy in persons without gonadal dysgenesis[9] although the possibility of this occurring by chance has not been entirely ruled out, and endometrial cancer is known to be associated with feminizing tumors of the ovaries.[10,11,12]

Finally, the question arises as to the pathogenesis of tumors in daughters whose mothers took estrogens during pregnancy. Herbst et al[13] in screening 34 teenage and young adult women who had been exposed to stilbestrol in utero, found that 13 had vaginal adenosis (glandular epithelium in the vagina),

21 had cervical erosion (glandular epithelium in the portio of the cervix) and 7 had transverse cervical or vaginal ridges (partial septa). These investigators provide evidence that the adenosis is of congenital, probably Müllerian, in origin. In addition, adenocarcinomas of the vagina have been observed in close proximity to adenosis. It appears, therefore, that the stilbestrol acted as a teratogen in addition to being a carcinogen. This possibility is supported by first trimester initiation of stilbestrol therapy by all mothers of the patients reported here.

REFERENCES

1. P. Greenwald, J.J. Barlow, P.C. Nasca and W.S. Burnett, *N. Engl. J. Med.* *285*, 390, 1971.

2. A.L. Herbst and R.E. Scully, *Cancer 25*, 745, 1970.

3. A.L. Herbst, H. Ulfelder and D.C. Poskanzer, *N. Engl. J. Med. 284*, 878, 1971.

4. P. Shubik and J.L. Hartwell, *in* U.S. Dept. Health, Educ. Welfare, Public Health Service Public. No. 149, Suppl. 2, 127, 1969.

5. F.J. Rauscher, *in* DES Hearings, U.S. Senate, Subcommittee on Health, July 20, 1972.

6. P. Greenwald, P.C. Nasca, W.S. Burnett and A.K. Polan, *Cancer* (in press).

7. K.L. Noller, D.G. Decker, A.P. Lanier and L.T. Kurland, *Mayo Clin. Proc. 47*, 629, 1972.

8. B.S. Cutler, A.P. Forbes, F.M. Ingersoll and R.E. Scully, *N. Engl. J. Med. 287*, 628, 1972.

9. A. Vass, *Am. J. Obst. Gynec. 58*, 748, 1949.

10. R.M. Corbet and W.H. Tod, *J. Obst. Gynec. Brit. Emp. 59*, 368, 1952.

11. L.A. Emge, *Obst. & Gynec. 1*, 511, 1953.

12. B.B. Silverman, R.T. O'Neill and J.J. Mikuta, *Surg. Gynec. & Obst. 134*, 244, 1972.

13. A.L.Herbst, R.J.Kurman and R.E.Scully, *Obst. & Gynec. 40*, 287, 1972.

PERINATAL MORTALITY, RACE, SOCIAL STATUS AND HOSPITAL OF BIRTH: THE ASSOCIATION WITH BIRTHWEIGHT

David Rush

Among firstborns in Aberdeen, Scotland, low birthweight varied by social status, but perinatal mortality among low birthweight infants of different classes was nearly the same (Table 1).[1] The rate of low birthweight for women of lowest social status was 10%, nearly double that of women of highest social status. However, the range of perinatal mortality among infants born under 2500 grams was only 15% (21.9% to 25.1% mortality). Shapiro et al.[2] have shown that although American black perinatal mortality is nearly double that of whites, the risk of mortality at given birthweights for the two races shows slight advantage for blacks to 2500 grams, and a marked disadvantage only over that weight. That the risk of perinatal death is well expressed by birthweight, has recently been reiterated by our group, for several large populations, using sophisticated statistical techniques.[3]

Social status, and other maternal characteristics, generate the birthweight distribution of a population, and thus most of the risk of perinatal mortality. What group risks might there be, independent of birthweight? In this presentation we use the technique of direct adjustment to compare the risk of perinatal mortality independent of birthweight, between races, and among social strata and hospitals of delivery. Deviations in adjusted mortality should measure other risks, such as the technical quality of perinatal care. The Monroe County, New York region, from which these data originated, seemed an ideal area for such a study; the population was well-defined geographically, had a range of social status, the number of hospitals was limited, nearly all births took place in hospitals, few women went elsewhere for delivery, and the overall quality of data reporting was believed to be high. Of the seven hospitals in the county with obstetric services, six are urban (hospitals A through F, Table 2) and one rural (hospital G). Hospitals A through E are all large, general voluntary hospitals, while hospital F is a small proprietary hospital, primarily staffed by general practitioners, and without an accredited obstetric training program.

161

TABLE 1

10,724 First Births, Aberdeen, Scotland; From Thomson[1]

	HUSBANDS' SOCIAL CLASS		
	I–II	III	IV–V
No. of Births	1566	6801	2357
Birthweight 2500 grams, %	5.4	6.7	10.0
Perinatal Mortality Among Low Birthweight, %	24.4	25.1	21.9

METHODS

Through the generosity of the Monroe County Health Department, we were given access to all county birth certificates from December 1961, the time when they were first coded and punched on IBM computer cards, through either 1966 or 1967, depending on the analysis.

Unfortunately, gestation was not yet reported on the basis of the date of last menstrual period. (This improvement in reporting took place in January, 1968.) Neonatal deaths were identified through the file of Dr. Charles Odoroff, of the Monroe County Psychiatric Case Registry, we were able to use a computer program which translated addresses from the birth and death certificates into census tracts. Census tracts had previously been ranked into social strata, by income and other indices. This stratification had been developed for the Register.[4] Only birthweights of at least 1 lb. (454 grams), and only those certificates in which birthweight had been recorded, were included. This only slightly under-represented fetal mortality rates, but should not have introduced biases among groups. Children were classified as black if either parent was black. Adjustment for birthweight was by the direct method, by half pound groupings, using as the reference population the total cohort of live births during the period.

RESULTS AND DISCUSSION: HOSPITAL OF BIRTH, AND RACE

In Table 2a are the crude perinatal mortality rates by hospital and by race for the period through 1966. The black rate is nearly 70% higher than that of whites (39.2 versus 23.2 per thousand live births). Among hospitals, for whites (for whom larger numbers yield more stable rates), there is a low of 16.8 to a high of 27.8 perinatal deaths per thousand. Among the five large urban hospitals, the rates varied from 21.6 to 26.3 per thousand, a range of 22%.

In Table 2b are the birthweight adjusted perinatal mortality rates. The adjusted rate for blacks is lower than that for whites, and the range of variation among the five urban general hospitals narrows, to a range of 9% (Table 2b). The high rates of hospital F were not explained by a disadvantageous distribution of birthweight in its population, nor were the low rates of hospital G explained away entirely by its advantageous distribution of birthweight. These data do suggest that most of the differences in perinatal mortality among the five general urban hospitals had to do with the birthweight distribution of the infants born here, rather than any differences in the perinatal care. We can only speculate on the divergent rates for hospitals F and G.

163

TABLE 2a

Perinatal Mortality, per 1000 Live Births, by Hospital and Race, Monroe County, New York, December 1961 – 1966

	HOSPITAL							Home Delivery	TOTAL
	A	B	C	D	E	F	G		
WHITE									
Live Births (n)	8662	11637	14217	11892	12138	1332	3042	100	63020
Fetal Mortality[1]	13.0	10.8	10.8	10.0	12.2	12.0	9.2	90.0	11.3
Neonatal Mortality[2]	13.3	11.3	12.2	13.6	9.4	15.8	7.6	80.0	11.9
Perinatal Mortality[3]	26.3	22.1	23.0	23.6	21.6	27.8	16.8	170.0	23.2
BLACK									
Live Births (n)	3654	282	719	1297	666	43	78	29	6768
Fetal Mortality	17.2	21.3	16.7	10.0	19.5	23.3	12.8	206.9	17.0
Neonatal Mortality	19.4	31.9	22.3	24.7	28.5	23.3	0	69.0	22.0
Perinatal Mortality	36.6	53.2	39.0	34.7	48.0	46.6	12.8	275.9	39.2

[1] Fetal mortality = all fetal deaths, at least one pound birthweight/1000 live births.
[2] Neonatal mortality = all deaths under 28 days of life/1000 live births.
[3] Perinatal mortality = fetal mortality and neonatal mortality.

TABLE 2b

Perinatal Mortality, per 1000 Live Births, Directly Adjusted for Birthweight, by Hospital and Race, Monroe County, New York, December 1961 – 1966

	HOSPITAL							Home Delivery	TOTAL
	A	B	C	D	E	F	G		
WHITE									
Fetal Mortality[1]	13.4	12.1	11.6	10.1	13.9	12.7	10.5	11.6	12.1
Neonatal Mortality[2]	12.9	12.9	13.6	14.0	11.3	16.3	10.4	20.6	13.0
Perinatal Mortality[3]	26.3	25.0	25.2	24.1	25.2	29.0	20.9	32.2	25.1
BLACK									
Fetal Mortality	12.0	13.2	11.6	7.1	9.1	—[4]	—[4]	—[4]	11.2
Neonatal Mortality	12.9	12.1	14.2	14.4	12.9	—[4]	—[4]	—[4]	13.3
Perinatal Mortality	24.9	25.3	25.8	21.5	22.0	—[4]	—[4]	—[4]	24.5

[1] Fetal mortality = all fetal deaths, at least one pound birthweight/per 1000 live births.
[2] Neonatal mortality = all deaths under 28 days of life/1000 live births.
[3] Perinatal mortality = fetal mortality and neonatal mortality.
[4] Under 100 live births.

SOCIAL STATUS

Among questions raised by the above data was whether differences in mortality by race could be explained by differences in social status. In Table 3 are presented mean birthweight and mean length of gestation by race (for a slightly different cohort of women; it also includes those delivering in 1967). There was no gradient for gestation by social status among whites, but there probably was among blacks. (The data on gestation must be interpreted with caution.) However, there were very few black infants born to women residing in more affluent areas (strata I and II). Those that did had longer gestations, similar to white women living in the same areas. There were birthweight gradients among whites and blacks by social status; the gradient among whites was about 60 grams, and among blacks, about double that. Some, but not all of the racial disparity in birthweight is accounted for by comparing women living in similar socio-economic areas. The overall birthweight difference between races was 216 grams; the average difference within census tract ranks was reduced to 153 grams. The reported mean white gestation was .4 weeks longer; within census tract rankings, .26 weeks.

The social status ranking procedure was unlikely to have comparable meaning in the two races. However, within the races, the ranking probably was capable of scaling, so much so that, on the average, women in one group would be generally better off than those ranked below. Thus, we can conclude that some of the differences between the races for birthweight, and probably for gestation were due to social status; whether all the racial difference can be attributed to the lower social status of blacks cannot be solved until we have a scheme that can rank women by social class, independent of race, which we do not have.

Crude perinatal mortality varied dramatically by social status for whites (Table 4). The rate for the lowest social rank (32.8/1000) was 65% higher than that of the highest (19.9/1000). There was a regular gradient between these extremes. The effect was more extensive among males (80% excess; 40.1 versus 22.3/1000) than among females (46% excess; 25.6 versus 17.5/1000). This is consistent with increased male vulnerability to mortality to almost all causes at all ages (i.e., whatever the social or medical stresses that are operative, they are more operative among males).

The birthweight adjusted rates are far less disparate. Among white males, the rates are nearly identical for ranks I–IV; only the lowest rank showed a marked disadvantage (35.4/1000, versus rates from 28.4 to 30.8/1000 for the higher ranks). For females, ranks II–IV are similar; the highest rank has some advantages, and the lowest, only a slight disadvantage. The range narrows to 18.9/1000 to 24.5/1000, a difference of 30%.

166

TABLE 3

Birthweight and Gestation, by Race and Social Status, All Live Births, Monroe County, New York, December 1961 – 1967

Social Rank	WHITE			BLACK			Difference in mean birthweight, white-black
	Live Births, Number	Birthweight (grams)	Gestation (weeks)	Live Births, Number	Birthweight (grams)	Gestation (weeks)	
I	5,705	3297	39.7	20	3175	39.5	122
II	21,655	3305	39.6	90	3189	39.8	116
III	28,874	3283	39.6	769	3107	39.2	176
IV	9,108	3235	39.6	2,714	3067	39.1	168
V	2,908	3240	39.6	4,296	3059	39.2	181
UNKNOWN	4,621	3271	39.5	149	2999	39.1	272
TOTAL	72,971	3283	39.6	8,038	3067	39.2	216

(The average mean difference of birthweight between whites and blacks, within social groups, was 153 grams; of gestation, .26 weeks.)

TABLE 4

Perinatal Mortality, per 1000 Live Births, by Race, Sex and Social Rank, Directly Adjusted for Birthweight, Monroe County New York, December 1961–1967

SOCIAL RANK		WHITE			BLACK		
		MALE	FEMALE	TOTAL	MALE	FEMALE	TOTAL
I	Crude rate	22.3	17.5	19.9	–	–	–
	B.W. adjusted rate	29.3	18.9	24.2	–	–	–
	(n)*	(2,963)	(2,859)	(5,822)	(8)	(12)	(20)
II	Crude rate	22.3	19.8	21.1	–	45.5	21.7
	B.W. adjusted rate	28.4	22.6	25.6			
	(n)*	(11,382)	(10,738)	(22,120)	(48)	(44)	(92)
III	Crude rate	27.4	19.1	23.3	53.4	38.7	45.8
	B.W. adjusted rate	30.5	21.8	26.3	32.3	25.4	28.8
	(n)*	(15,277)	(14,291)	(29,568)	(393)	(413)	(806)
IV	Crude rate	30.7	25.9	28.4	49.6	39.8	44.7
	B.W. adjusted rate	30.8	22.9	27.0	25.9	25.8	25.8
	(n)*	(4,852)	(4,521)	(9,373)	(1,431)	(1,408)	(2,839)
V	Crude rate	40.1	25.6	32.8	42.3	32.1	37.2
	B.W. adjusted rate	35.4	24.5	29.9	27.5	20.3	23.9
	(n)*	(1,548)	(1,562)	(3,110)	(2,245)	(2,215)	(4,460)
UNKNOWN	(n)*	(2,345)	(2,335)	(4,680)	(63)	(89)	(152)
TOTAL	Crude rate	25.5	19.8	22.7	44.7	35.2	39.9
	B.W. adjusted rate	29.0	21.4	25.3	26.7	22.6	24.6
	(n)*	(38,366)	(36,303)	(74,669)	(4,186)	(4,181)	(8,367)

*(n) = live births

Thus, differences in the distribution of birthweight accounted for most of the variation in perinatal mortality among social strata for whites.

The risk of perinatal mortality associated with social status for whites that is independent of birthweight seems limited only to the extremes of status; some disadvantage for the lowest 4% or so of the population, and some advantage, for females only, in the highest stratum.

For blacks, the crude and adjusted rates vary inversely with social status, but numbers were small, and analyses need to be repeated with larger numbers.

CONCLUSION

In Monroe County, New York, for the period 1961–1967, differences in perinatal mortality between whites and blacks are entirely accounted for by differences in the birthweight distribution of the races. Among the five urban general hospitals of the area, the same is nearly true. For whites, most of the large gradient of perinatal mortality by social status is accounted for by birthweight distribution, with variation in perinatal mortality independent of birthweight limited to extremes of social status.

ACKNOWLEDGEMENTS

These data were collected while the author was associated with the Departments of Preventive Medicine and Pediatrics, University of Rochester School of Medicine. Drs. Wendell Ames and Margaret Rathbun, of the Monroe County Health Department, kindly made these data available. Programming and other assistance was supplied by Peter Fergus. Help from Dr. Charles Odoroff, and other staff of the Monroe County Psychiatric Case Registry, is gratefully acknowledged.

REFERENCES

1.   A.M. Thomson, *Mod. Probl. Pediat. 8,* 197, 1963.

2.   S. Shapiro, E.R. Schlesinger and R.E.L. Nesbitt, Jr., Infant, Perinatal, Maternal and Childhood Mortality in the United States, Harvard University Press, Cambridge, 1968.

3.   M. Susser, F.A. Marolla and J. Fleiss, *Am. J. Epidemiol. 96,* 197, 1972.

4.   H. Babigian and C. Odoroff, *Am. J. Psychiatry 126,* 470, 1969.

MATERNAL SMOKING DURING GESTATION AND INFANT MORPHOLOGIC VARIATION: PRELIMINARY REPORT CONCERNING BIRTH WEIGHT AND INCIDENCE OF TRANSVERSE PALMAR CREASES

E. B. Hook*, ***
S. Selvin**
J. Garfinkel*
M. Greenberg***

1. Introduction

The rationale for the initiation of the studies discussed here has been described at length elsewhere.[1] Briefly, the frequency of selected minor defects has been monitored in a local newborn population and some selected variables associated with pregnancy also recorded. The high frequency of some minor birth defects in the newborn population studied suggested these might be plausible markers for a pilot investigation of the subtle human teratogenicity of tobacco smoking. Furthermore, the data collected provided an additional opportunity to investigate some further aspects of the well known association of maternal tobacco smoking and low birth weight.

An ubiquitous environmental factor such as maternal smoking could have a relatively small teratogenic effect (perhaps producing no more than a maximum increase of 20–30% in the frequency of any *single* major defect) and yet result in a very large social burden because of the great number of individuals (i.e., fetuses) exposed. But detection of such an effect through investigation of rare defects might prove very difficult. However, investigation of markers detectable at birth which are relatively frequent and which are known to be associated with a deleterious phenotype, might be more productive.

2. Previous studies

The reports of the association of maternal tobacco smoking effect with

---

*Birth Defects Institute, New York State Department of Health.
**Department of Biostatistics, University of California, Berkeley.
***Department of Pediatrics, Albany Medical College of Union University.

lower birth weight have been numerous.[2] Every study to our knowledge has shown such an association. The effect appears to be primarily associated with growth retardation of the fetus. To our knowledge, there has not been, to date, any study well documenting a higher incidence of birth defects in infants of smoking mothers. (There have been conflicting reports concerning a possibly higher incidence of fetal loss and neonatal death in infants of smoking mothers, but we have not investigated this question. The evidence provided in a recent review[3] appears convincing concerning this association.)

3. Specific questions

As of August 15, 1972, we had extensive data on about 2,500 singleton, white infants without major congenital malformation who survived the neonatal period and were born in a particular 12 month period. (These infants were investigated during our ongoing monitoring program of minor birth defects.) This is the largest category in our sample and, therefore, we restrict this initial investigation to this group. We emphasize moreover, that the analysis presented here is a preliminary one. About six percent of the children in our sample had a single palmar flexion crease, hereafter referred to as a simian crease. This defect is the most frequent minor malformation we have detected and we have, therefore, limited the initial investigation to this malformation. Additional evidence from earlier studies of our own and others that suggested it was worth study were: (i) it tends to occur in association with such disorders as (a) isolated congenital heart disease, (b) idiopathic mental retardation, (c) multiple malformation syndromes; (ii) it can apparently be produced by known teratogens such as amethopterin, rubella and thalidomide; (iii) it exhibited a frequency correlated with birth weight, parental age and sex.[1]

Before investigating an association of maternal tobacco smoking with simian creases, however, we wished to be sure that the association with diminished birth weight reported by others existed in our own sample.

4. Birth weight

We looked at smoking habits during the second trimester. The results (Table 1) suggested that up to about 1 pack a day there was a strong "dose-response" curve but beyond that a leveling off. (There are relatively few individuals in each of the smoking categories so, in presenting some of the data below, we have pooled all those smokers who smoked less than one pack per day, denoting them as "light" smokers, and all those smoking one or more packs per day as "heavy" smokers. Furthermore, we do not have all the information on each rubric for every infant in the study, so the data in particular tables will not always add up to the same total.) As other investigators had

TABLE 1
Birth Weights of Babies by 2nd Trimester Smoking Status

	non-smokers	smokers who stopped	< ½ pack/day	< 1 pack/day	< 1½ packs/day	< 2 packs/day	≥ 2 packs/day	Total
Total	1,351	102	220	280	409	122	103	2,587
Mean (lbs.)	7.62	7.64	7.40	7.16	7.03	7.01	6.98	7.40
S.D.	1.13	1.01	1.11	1.07	1.11	1.13	1.33	1.15
Males only	692	54	107	160	198	67	54	1,332
Mean (lbs.)	7.74	7.82	7.43	7.30	7.06	7.14	7.05	7.51
S.D.	1.14	0.97	1.20	1.04	1.24	1.10	1.52	1.19
Females only	659	48	113	120	211	55	49	1,255
Mean (lbs.)	7.48	7.43	7.37	6.98	7.01	6.85	6.90	7.29
S.D.	1.11	1.03	1.01	1.07	0.97	1.14	1.09	1.10

found, this effect could not be attributed to concomitant variation of maternal smoking with socioeconomic status (at lease as measured in our study by years of schooling of the mother), maternal age, parity or height. Since tobacco smoking is correlated with coffee drinking as well as ingestion of some types of alcoholic beverages, and to our knowledge these latter factors had not been studied by others who had looked at birth weight, we investigated these specific factors as well. Our initial results indicated that coffee drinking did not appear responsible for the observed tobacco smoking effect (Table 2). Analysis of alcohol consumption is difficult since one must distinguish at a minimum, the form in which it is ingested (beer, wine or "other spirits"), the average frequency of ingestion and the maximum amount likely to be ingested at any specific occasion. There is the additional problem of variation of these ingestion patterns with time. At this point, we will say only that stratifying on the single alcohol variable which gave the greatest negative correlation with birth weight (and even this was of borderline significance), the association of low birth weight with maternal tobacco smoking was undiminished (see Table 3). One other observation of interest concerns mothers who smoked during the early part of gestation but then stopped. In our own small sample of children of about 100 mothers who smoked at some time during the first trimester but not during the second, the mean birth weight was about the same as those children of mothers who did not smoke at all (see Table 1).

5. Simian creases

We distinguish types of abnormal palmar creases by their variation in intensity from a full simian (i.e., single transverse palmar flexion crease with no branches) to "bridged" creases of various sorts. For the purposes of this initial analysis we will ignore these gradients, as well as the question of laterality. An individual with a unilateral bridged crease will be considered with weight equal to that of an individual with bilateral full simian creases. (With collection of additional data, of course, we hope to be able to analyze factors associated with variation in the expression of the trait. A description of the exact diagnostic features used is in preparation and will appear elsewhere.)

Some of the factors associated with the incidence trait in newborns are summarized in Tables 4A and 4B. It can be seen that there is a positive association with male sex, presence of simian crease in the mother and number of years of schooling of the mother *in children born to mothers who do not smoke*. ("Non-smokers" were those who had not smoked in the year before birth of the child.) The palmar creases are heavily influenced by flexion movements of the hands between the 7th and 14th week of development.[4] A case could be made for analyzing the association of this defect in the infant with

174

TABLE 2

Mean Birth Weight by Maternal Coffee Ingestion and Tobacco Smoking

	COFFEE CONSUMPTION		
SMOKING	None	Some 2 cups/day	3–40 cups/day
None	N = 529 M = 7.69 lbs. S.D. = 1.10	N = 664 M = 7.61 lbs. S.D. = 1.13	N = 158 M = 7.41 S.D. = 1.14 lbs.
"Light"	N = 152 M = 7.44 lbs. S.D. = 1.17	N = 210 M = 7.30 lbs. S.D. = 1.13	N = 138 M = 7.02 lbs. S.D. = 1.03
"Heavy"	N = 154 M = 7.03 lbs. S.D. = 1.20	N = 212 M = 7.17 lbs. S.D. = 1.08	N = 268 M = 6.89 lbs. S.D. = 1.11

TABLE 3

Birth Weight by Maternal Tobacco Smoking and Maximum Beer Consumption/Occasion

	BEER CONSUMPTION		
	None	< 2 pints	> 2 pints
None	N = 974 M = 7.63 S.D. = 1.10	N = 233 M = 7.57 S.D. = 1.17	N = 144 M = 7.65 S.D. = 1.21
S M O K I N G "Light"	N = 335 M = 7.28 S.D. = 1.12	N = 71 M = 7.26 S.D. = 1.11	N = 94 M = 7.23 S.D. = 1.30
"Heavy"	N = 403 M = 7.09 S.D. = 1.05	N = 85 M = 6.95 S.D. = 1.30	N = 146 M = 6.85 S.D. = 1.21

*Comment: Of all six "alcohol" variables examined (average daily frequency and maximum intake on single occasion for wine, beer and "other spirits"), the maximum intake of beer had the lowest correlation (i.e. the greatest negative correlation) with birth weight (-.04). (The value for the others varied from +.01 to -.02, the latter for average frequency for beer intake.) Maximum beer intake also had the highest positive correlation with tobacco smoking (+.14). The value for the others varied from -.10 to +.08, the latter for mean beer intake. The correlation of mean beer intake and maximum beer intake was +.67. A correlation coefficient of +.05 or greater (or -.05 or less) for these data is different from zero at the 95% level.

176

TABLE 4A

Incidence of Simian Creases in Study*

Male Infants	101/1329	= 7.6%
Female Infants	58/1256	= 4.6%
Mothers	91/2576	= 3.5%

*Comment: Data were not available on all mothers. The difference in frequency between daughters may reflect (a) diminished fitness associated with the presence of a simian crease in females, and/or (b) a change with age in appearance of the crease, and/or (c) temporal changes in incidence of the crease over the last 20–30 years. Other evidence (see 1 for references) suggests that a) accounts for at least part of the difference.

TABLE 4B

Simian Crease in Infants Born to *Non-smoking* Mothers

1. By sex (non-smoking mothers)

	Male	Female
n	692	659
frequency with simian crease	7.4%	4.3%

2. By presence of maternal crease pattern (non-smoking mothers)

	Infants born to mothers *with* simian crease	Infants born to mothers *without* simian crease
n	47	1300
frequency with simian crease	14.9%	5.5%

3. By years of schooling of mother (non-smoking mothers)

	≤11 years	> 12 years	12 years
n	168	533	645
frequency with simian crease	7.1%	6.4%	4.8%

either the second trimester or first trimester smoking habit of the mother. (It might seem first trimester patterns would be the most logical to use, but our coding was for the *maximum* daily amount smoked in each three month period. What changes that occurred in smoking habits during first trimester were often just after the mother discovered she was pregnant, before the 7th week. She may have then lowered her smoking frequency, but would have been coded as smoking the earlier, higher amount for this trimester. If her pattern was subsequently constant (as it frequently was), the amount coded in second trimester would be more likely to reflect the exposure during the postulated critical period.

In Table 5 appears the relationship of simian creases in infants to the second trimester smoking habits of their mothers. Table 6 provides the same analysis for the first trimester. In the rest of this discussion, we shall be dealing only with second trimester smoking habits.

The distribution of simian creases among non-smokers, "light" smokers and "heavy" smokers appears unlikely due to chance (chi^2 = 9.49, d.f. = 2, $p < .01$). The cell which contributes the greatest amount to the value of chi^2 is that for a "heavy" smoker. (For the comparison of heavy smokers and non-smokers, chi^2 = 4.35, d.f. = 1, $p < .05$.) The difference between infants of non-smokers and heavy smokers is present whether we stratify on height, years of schooling of mother, maternal age of mother, presence of crease in mother, birth order, coffee drinking patterns in the mother or alcohol ingestion. With regard to the relationship of birth weight and simian crease there is an interesting sex difference. The mean birth weight of males with simian creases born to non-smoking mothers (7.73 lbs.) is slightly less than that of males with normal creases born to non-smokers (7.75 lbs.) but the mean birth weight of males with simian creases born to heavy smokers (6.59 lbs.) is markedly less than that of males with normal creases born to heavy smokers (7.13 lbs.). In females, however, the birth weights appear relatively independent of the presence of a simian crease, when the categories are stratified by maternal heavy smoker status. (The values are 7.46 vs. 7.49 and 6.97 vs. 6.96 respectively.) But when we stratify by absolute birth weight in each smoking category, it may be seen that for both sexes there is a greater frequency of simian creases in children of mothers who smoke heavily in each birth weight category (Table 7). This suggests but does not yet establish that the association of simian creases and maternal smoking is not simply a result of the effect of smoking upon birth weight. We emphasize, however, that more data must be collected and more extensive analysis done before firm conclusions are possible about the nature of the relationship and interdependent associations of birth weight, simian creases and maternal tobacco smoking.

The fact that slightly fewer simian creases are observed in children of light

179

TABLE 5

Distribution of Simian Creases Among Babies by Second Trimester Smoking Status of Their Mothers

	Non-smokers	"light" smokers		"heavy" smokers			Total
		< ½ pack/day	< 1 pack/day	< 1½ packs/day	< 2 packs/day	> 2 packs/day	
Number	79/1351	7/220	13/278	33/409	9/122	11/104	152/2484
Frequency of infants with simian creases	5.9%	3.2%	4.7%	8.1%	7.4%	10.6%	6.1%
		4.0%			8.3%		

*Those who had not smoked in the year prior to birth of the child. Those who smoked in first trimester but stopped completely are excluded in this analysis.

180

TABLE 6

Distribution of Simian Creases Among Babies by First Trimester Smoking Status of Their Mothers

	Non-smokers*	"light" smokers			"heavy" smokers		Total
		<½ pack/day	<1 pack/day	<1½ packs/day	<2 packs/day	≥2 packs/day	
Number	79/1351	7/224	17/280	34/473	11/126	10/112	158/2566
Frequency of infants with simian creases	5.9%	3.1%	6.1%	7.2%	8.7%	8.9%	6.2%

*Those who had not smoked in the year prior to the birth of the child.

TABLE 7

The Frequency of Infants with Simian Creases, by Birth Weight Category

BIRTH WEIGHT

	less than 6 lbs.	6.00 – 6.99 lbs.	7.00 – 7.99 lbs.	8 lbs. or more
Female infants born to non-smokers	2/45 = 4.4%	5/156 = 3.9%	9/242 = 3.7%	11/216 = 5.1%
Female infants born to "heavy" smokers	4/48 = 8.3%	8/107 = 7.5%	6/110 = 5.2%	3/44 = 6.8%
Male infants born to non-smokers	5/40 = 12.5%	5/109 = 4.6%	23/265 = 8.7%	18/278 = 6.5%
Male infants born to "heavy" smokers	10/55 = 18.2%	6/84 = 7.1%	10/106 = 9.4%	6/74 = 8.1%

smokers than non-smokers indicates why some caution is necessary in evaluating the opposite but stronger trend in children of heavy smokers. The difference between children of non-smokers and light smokers is not "significant". (chi^2 = 2.05, d.f. = 1, p = .15) Nevertheless, the trend appears relatively consistent when we stratify on sex and a number of other variables; e.g., birth order, maternal age, coffee drinking, etc. (Only among children born to mothers with a greater than 12th grade education is there a greater frequency of simian creases in children of light smokers than non-smokers.) The trend is strongest (that is, the incidence of simian creases is least) in children of those light smoking mothers who have smoked less than a half a pack a day. This category includes all mothers who have smoked between one cigarette in three months and nine cigarettes per day. Thus, it is the most heterogeneous group in our sample in terms of smoking exposure. We have looked for some consistent way in which this group differs from non-smokers and heavy smokers, but have not yet been successful. An alternative explanation is that there is some agent or pattern associated with both non-smoking and a higher incidence of simian creases. But if there is some such factor it does not appear to be associated with a birth weight effect since the mean birth weight of children of light smokers is lower than that of children of non-smokers. Alternatively, the observation may be due to "chance".

Hopefully, collection of further data and more refined analysis of smoking patterns in this group will allow closer scrutiny of these trends.

CONCLUSION

A preliminary analysis of data collected in the course of an ongoing investigation of maternal smoking and newborn morphological variation has been presented. The association of maternal smoking with diminished infant birth weight found by others is confirmed here and it is shown that this effect cannot be attributed to association of cigarette smoking with coffee or alcoholic beverage ingestion. There is a trend to a higher incidence of simian creases in infants born to mothers who are heavy smokers than in infants born to non-smokers (or light smokers) which cannot be explained by the lower birth weight of infants of heavy smokers but, at this point, it would be premature to suggest that maternal smoking is the causal factor for this difference.

ACKNOWLEDGEMENTS

The data has been gathered by a number of individuals including: Carol Winkler, Marguerite Linda Powers, Mary Beth Hanner, Susan Denise Brown, Grace Conway, Sandra Loomis, Jeanne Baum, Jane Garvey, Peggy Aldrich and Ellen Desmond. Miss Aldrich and Mrs. Desmond, in addition, greatly assisted with some of the tabulations. We thank Sister Jean McGinty, Dr. Allan MacCollam and other members of the staff at St. Peter's Hospital for their cooperation, as well as the members of the staff at Albany Medical Center Hospital. Dr. R. Korns advised on the original plan of this study. The programming was done by K. Mohlman and R. Hughes. This study was aided by a grant from the American Medical Association Education and Research Foundation and, in addition, by a grant from the National Institute for Child Health and Human Development.

REFERENCES

1. E.B. Hook, *in* Monitoring, Birth Defects and Environment, E.B. Hook, D.T. Janerich and I.H. Porter (Eds.), Academic Press, New York, p. 177, 1971.

2. P.S. Larson and H. Silvette, *in* Tobacco Experimental and Clinical Studies (Supplement II), Williams and Wilkins, Baltimore, 1971.

3. D. Rush and E.H. Kass, *Amer. J. Epidemiol. 96,* 183, 1972.

4. G.A. Popich and D.W. Smith, *J. Pediat. 77,* 1017, 1970.

IMPERFECT POTATO AND SPINA BIFIDA

James H. Renwick

THE PROBLEM

Spina bifida, anencephaly and certain types of hydrocephaly constitute one of the commonest major malformation classes in the United States: at least 1 per 1,000 total births; at least 5,000 per year. Many children with spina bifida now survive crippled and incontinent.

THE CLAIM

That 96 percent of the anencephaly and spina bifida (and some of the hydrocephaly) in Britain and countries with similar dietary customs, is preventable by avoidance of specific but unidentified substances in certain (diseased or damaged) potato tubers, during the first month of pregnancy and the preceding month.[1] An equal number of pregnancies now miscarried would be expected to be carried to full term on the same regimen.

The claim is put in the abative rather than the causative mode primarily for testability and for clarity of communication. We would not be allowed to test a causal claim.

THE EVIDENCE

Three separate relationships between the quality of potatoes and the incidence of ASB (anencephaly or spina bifida):

Seasonal

Damage done particularly in May (very early in pregnancy) when, in Britain, the old potatoes are at their worst quality (after winter storage). In the United States, potatoes are obtainable fresh all year round from some state or other so there is less need to store potatoes. Those that are stored are stored under near-optimal conditions, hence the seasonal effect on ASB incidence is not much in evidence in the United States.

185

Geographical

Relationship between severity of late blight (*Phytophthora infestans*) infection in a region and the local ASB incidence rate; e.g., Maine has more blight and more ASB than Idaho; Ireland has more blight and more ASB than eastern England. (The rate in Belfast and Dublin has been one percent at times.)

Year-to-Year

The claims made on the basis of the above relationships. The obvious prediction was then made that a blight year would be followed, at a suitable interval for winter storage of potatoes and maturation of the developing fetus, by an outbreak of spina bifida births. This prediction was validated repeatedly by collating the potato literature and the ASB medical literature.[2,3,4,5]

MONKEY EXPERIMENTS

At my suggestion, Professor David E. Poswillo[6] has fed marmoset monkeys with a preparation of blighted potato before and during early pregnancy. He obtained four osseous defects of the skull out of eleven offspring, and no such defects in the eleven controls (or 80 previous marmoset young in his colony).

The evidence, therefore, comes mainly from blight but there are thirty or so other afflictions of the potato. The *claim*, therefore, does not mention blight.

POSSIBLE MECHANISM

Epidemiological evidence suggests that it is the antibiotic or phytoalexin response of the potato to infection or injury that is to be avoided by women. Rishitin, rishitinol, lubimin, phytuberin, the solanines and chaconines are some of the known anti-fungal agents in potato that might be investigated in the marmoset model for the anti-embryo role. Plant breeders may have inadvertently increased the teratogenic potential of some potato varieties while breeding for resistance to fungi such as blight and wart.

GUIDANCE

Despite our present ignorance of the nature of the teratogens in potatoes and their routes of absorption by women in early pregnancy, the evidence on preventability is good and already sufficient to allow guidance to be given.[7]

If a woman in her reproductive years wishes to reduce her chance of giving birth to a child with a major malformation of the central nervous system, she should avoid all contact with imperfect potatoes, at least during the first four weeks of pregnancy (when she may not know she is pregnant) and in the preceding four weeks. The whole of a potato should be discarded if any part of it is discolored, greened, diseased, sprouted, scabbed, cut, bruised, holed or in any other way imperfect, as the antibiotics that the diseased potato synthesizes and that are to be avoided are present also in the apparently healthy part of the potato. To minimize absorption by inhalation or through the skin she should, whenever possible, also avoid potato-steam and wear gloves while peeling and handling potatoes.

FURTHER WORK

Potato-avoidance trial among high-risk women (with ASB child already), to establish the claim. Identification of teratogens and their main routes of entry.

REFERENCES

1. J.H. Renwick, *Brit. J. prev. soc. Med. 26,* 67, 1972.

2. J.H. Renwick, *Lancet 2,* 336, 1972.

3. J.H. Renwick, *New Scientist 56,* 277, 1972.

4. J.H. Renwick, *Lancet 2,* 967, 1972.

5. J.H. Renwick, *New Society 22,* 212, 1972.

6. D.E. Poswillo, D. Sopher and S. Mitchell, *Nature 239,* 462, 1972.

7. J.H. Renwick, *Brit. J. orev. soc. Med. 26,* 269, 1972.

DISCUSSION

DR. LILIENFELD: The paper by Dr. Renwick is most interesting and I guess after seeing that monkey, I'm all in favor of high quality potatoes. Dr. Renwick has challenged us, however, to produce a mother of an anencephalic who has not eaten potatoes. At the moment, your data is based upon correlations between the frequency of blight in different areas and the frequency of anencephaly. Have you looked at the frequency of potato consumption among mothers who have anencephalic children, in contrast to a control group of mothers?

DR. RENWICK: Dr. Lilienfeld, I would like to do a study on potato avoidance. In other words, this would be a prospective study of the type you're suggesting. On the other hand, I would not like to do a retrospective study of potato consumption because it is not possible to assess potato quality even when you have the potatoes available. It is certainly impossible to assess it nine months previously. And so, I feel retrospective studies are a waste of time. We need an immediate potato-avoidance trial of high risk women – those who have already had one such malformation – and, therefore, have a 5% risk of having another. In Britain, this would be perfectly feasible on a national scale in two or three years.

DR. SHAPIRO: As far as the empiric risk figures for recurrence of anencephaly, would you say that if you could remove whatever it is that happens to the potato and causes anencephaly, that the risk figure would then increase and you'd have a second type of anencephaly with a possibly greater recurrence risk? Is this recurrence risk based upon eating potatoes? In other words, is there a 5% chance that if you eat a potato again you're going to have an anencephalic – or are there two types of anencephaly, one of which is based upon consumption of the blighted potato?

DR. RENWICK: Let me answer this question as to whether we can assume the potato avoidance regime would be equally effective in the familial cases as in the sporadic cases. I'm assuming that all women are not susceptible to whatever it is. There are presumably either acquired or genetic susceptibility factors. If it were acquired it could be, for instance, bacterial fluid which could detoxify or affect the absorption of a teratogen. I think potato avoidance would lower the 5% risk to very near zero. Thus, I would suspect that the trial would be quite feasible because numbers would be quite practical.

MRS. GREEN: Dr. Renwick, the border between Poland and Russia is moist and has a high potato consumption and, at least at one time, had a large Jewish population which has a low incidence of anencephaly. How do you explain these data?

DR. RENWICK: The comparison between the quality of potatoes eaten in one country and the quality of potatoes eaten in another is difficult. The Poles have their own varieties of potato that are not known for having specialized blight resistance. In other words, they have not made a great effort to get the potato to defend itself with antibiotics. Therefore, their potatoes, perhaps, are still fairly harmless. The habits of how you deal with blighted potatoes are so different from one country to another and even from one class to another, that detailed explanation between countries is hopeless.

MRS. GREEN: Dr. Hook, the dermatoglyphics of the simian crease as well as the dermal ridges are considered to be dominant with reduced penetrance and inherited through both the mother and the father. Did you include fathers in your studies?

DR. HOOK: We are well aware of the significance of paternal genetic factors. The problem in these types of studies is one of ascertainment. It is easy to interview mothers in hospitals. They are very cooperative. But fathers are either not present, or when present, are immensely suspicious of questions relating to traits in them which we are investigating in their infants. In separate studies we are, in fact, seeking out normal males as propositi with simian creases and doing family studies where possible.

DR. HOOK: Dr. Renwick, if you advise avoidance of contact with potatoes, do you mean avoidance of every environment in which potatoes may exist, such as supermarkets or grocery stores where they are stored in bins? Furthermore, what about processed potatoes? In our society there is a great deal of exposure to potato chips, fried potatoes bought commercially and similar food items. Clearly, the consumer doesn't know the origins of potatoes in these products. Has the problem of blight been removed in their preparation?

DR. RENWICK: I think these compounds may well be volatile in steam but very unlikely to constitute a hazard in supermarkets where, in any case, the potatoes are usually enclosed in bags. I think the chance that there is enough in the atmosphere of supermarkets is negligible.

The question of the processed potato is interesting. In this country the incidence of malformation of the neural tube has been falling since 1932, and is still falling. In Europe it has been falling since about 1935, except for one epidemic in the 1950's which ended in 1960. Since then — this is unpublished data of a general practitioner in Rugby, England — it has been falling in about five different European countries that he has observed since 1960. Both these decreases are consistent with improved control of potato disease and better storage conditions (few are now stored outdoors and more are stored in air-conditioned rooms) but it also may be related to the increase in consumption of processed potatoes. Details of what goes on in the processing plants are not usually available but I do know that, for commercial reasons, these firms do provide extremely good storage conditions for their potatoes and they have very competent people looking after their potatoes.

One small issue which may be relevant is that one firm in Britain has assessed the rishitin level of its output and it's ten to the minus or less, so whatever goes into the potato is either safe already or its rishitin is destroyed during processing. It is too early to say as yet, but the rishitin is not there.

DR. NANCE: Dr. Renwick, would you comment on the concordance data on monozygotic twins with respect to your hypothesis. It seems to me that if the genotype of the mother or the fetus or the environment is important, one would expect a high concordance rate in MZ twins.

DR. RENWICK: I think the evidence is fairly clear that the concordance rate in MZ twins is not much higher, if any higher, than that in dizygotic twins which really means that the fetal genotype has very little influence on the outcome. The mother's genotype and the mother's environment are completely unresolvable and you can't resolve one from the other in some twins. You're presumably asking how I account for lower concordance rates and in my paper I gave two alternative explanations. I don't know which is correct. One is that the window through which the teratogen acts — the time window — is so short that some particular chemical process either does not occur or does occur according to chance factors. This would account for it. The other alternative method to account for it is to note that even mono-zygotic twins do not develop at exactly the same rate.

DR. RUSH: Dr. Renwick, I would like to know whether the form of potato that we're familiar with is the one that you've implicated. There are, of course, cultural uses of potato. There are populations in Africa which use tubers as a major source of calories and others which never use them at all and I would have thought that the epidemiology of the malformation (if these other tubers are susceptible to the diseases in question) should show striking

191

point-to-point variation by groups, depending on their diet staples. Do you have any data on this?

DR. RENWICK: The data from Africa are rather difficult to interpret. But, in Uganda, the incidence of these malformations is very low and they don't apparently have many potatoes. There is no blight on that side. In parts of Nigeria there is blight, but the consumption of potatoes is very low and, as has been pointed out to me in *The Lancet* in a notation by an anonymous critic, the figures for Nigeria are somewhat higher than would fit my theory in its simplest form. I don't pretend to know the explanation. It may be that the Nigerian data indicates that one of these teratogens may just possibly be present in another plant, but the tubers which Dr. Rush referred to in Nigeria are yams. I understand that these are not solaninacious plants and, therefore, not likely candidates.

I say that there are two teratogens — one for anencephaly and one for spina bifida following anencephaly and *vice versa*. In other words, there is a tendency for specificity of recurrence. This is even more marked in the twin data where you have a four to one excess of like over unlike pairs, when the twins are concordant, as they occasionally are. But, incident to these two teratogens, I am assuming both to be packaged in the potato and in fairly constant proportions and both switched on, like all these antibiotics, by the same stimuli.

SECTION V

SECTION V

PRESENT GUIDELINES FOR TERATOGENIC STUDIES IN EXPERIMENTAL ANIMALS

Frances O. Kelsey

The Food and Drug Administration has for some time recognized the hazards to the developing fetus of environmental chemicals including food additives, pesticides, cosmetics and drugs to which the pregnant mother may be exposed. The present discussion will consist of a brief review of the evolution of the Administration's policies with regard to screening for terato-genesis, a description in some detail of the teratology and other reproduction tests currently required for investigational new drugs and a consideration of the relevance of animal reproductive studies in assessing the safety of drugs in human beings.

In describing the evolution of the Food and Drug Administration's policy in screening of drugs for teratogenicity, it is necessary to review very briefly the federal laws relative to the introduction of new drugs in this country. The Pure Food and Drug Act of 1906 did little but prohibit the introduction into interstate commerce of adulterated and misbranded drugs. Manufacturers could introduce a drug at will. The onus rested on the government to produce evidence of adulteration or misbranding before a dangerous or ineffective drug could be withdrawn from the market. Repeated attempts to strengthen the 1906 Act failed until 1937 when approximately 100 persons died from a marketed drug that had as a solvent the toxic diethylene glycol.[1] It was clearly evident that little or no attempt had been made to determine the safety of this dosage form prior to its introduction. Recognition of this fact was the precipitating factor that lead to the passage of the 1938 Food, Drug and Cosmetic Act which, amongst other provisions, contained the so-called New Drug Provisions specifically directed towards insuring the safety of new drugs.

Under these provisions, a new drug could not be released for interstate commerce for other than investigational purposes until adequate evidence of its safety was presented to the Food and Drug Administration.

The required information presented in the form of a New Drug Application consisted of chemical control data, results of toxicity tests in animals, and of clinical trials in human subjects. Guidelines were developed by the Administration for the appropriate animal toxicity tests. Recommended procedures fell into reasonably well defined categories such as pharmacodynamics, acute toxicity, subacute toxicity, chronic toxicity, local external effects, and special studies which included reproduction. Thus, in a 1943 publication, reproduction tests were discussed as follows: "Reproduction studies are really a part of the chronic toxicity requirements and should yield information as to whether the substance in question will affect fertility, lactation, size of litter and mortality of the young."[2]

It should be noted there is no mention of teratology in the statement. However, at that time, congenital anomalies in animals were considered largely animal curiosities induced by dietary deficiencies or the occasional chemical, while in human beings these were generally ascribed to genetic influences with the possible exception of those associated with the history of exposure of the mother during pregnancy to x-radiation or to the German measles.

The first actual protocol proposed for reproduction tests by the Administration was designed to detect possible toxicity to food additives. This method is described in some detail in the publication issued in 1949 entitled "Procedures for the Appraisal of Toxicity of Chemicals in Foods". These guidelines were re-issued in 1955 and 1959 following certain revisions and modifications, including the extension of title and the contents to cover the appraisal of the safety of chemicals in drugs and cosmetics in addition to foods.[3]

The procedure recommended involved a three generation study in rats, with each group of rats being kept on the specific experimental diet throughout the test period. The 1959 revision of the brochure contained the statement, "Reproduction studies have assumed more importance in recent years. They are used whenever the chemical becomes a part of an important item of food, such as bread and milk, or may in any way affect the nutrition of the general population". The increasing importance was promoted in part by the additional safety requirements laid down by the Pesticides Amendments of 1959 and, a year later, by the Color Additives Amendments of 1960. Since 1963, three generation animal tests have been a requirement for establishing the tolerance level of pesticides.

Despite these guidelines it must be admitted, at least in hindsight, that many drugs entered the market between 1938 and 1962 with minimal evidence of safety in pregnancy. For example, the safety of a compound promoted amongst other things for nausea and vomiting of pregnancy, was supported by the claim that large doses of the drug had been given to a group of rats who throughout the period of study gave no evidence of abnormality

196

and bore normal litters. In actuality, this chronic toxicity study involved only 4 animals, 2 males and 2 females, who bore two litters each. The only data provided were animal weights. Clinical claims for safe use in pregnancy were based on two published reports involving a total of 132 women with nausea and vomiting of pregnancy. In no instance was the outcome of pregnancy reported.

Again, in the case of a drug advocated for treatment of threatened abortion, animal reproduction studies had not been done, although earlier, a chemically related compound had been reported to have a virilizing effect in offspring of rabbits receiving the drug during pregnancy. Clinical studies involved less than 25 patients. The outcome of pregnancy was not given in all cases but while some 14 live births were recorded, in no case was the sex of the child mentioned, let alone its condition at birth.

On the other hand, the abortifacient effects of aminopterin were noted in rats prior to the release of this drug to the market in 1951. The labeling on the container included a strong warning that the drug was only to be used in the treatment of acute leukemias in children and the package insert carried the additional information that "folic acid antagonists have been shown to have deleterious effect on the development of the embryo in experimental animals, hence they should never be used in pregnancy." The teratogenic effect of aminopterin on the human fetus was unfortunately subsequently demonstrated by reports of severely malformed children whose mothers had received aminopterin during pregnancy for therapeutic or criminal abortion.[4,5]

In 1960, when the application for Thalidomide was first submitted, the FDA had become much more alert to possible hazards of drugs to the fetus and the newborn. There was an increasing appreciation of the fact that virtually all drugs could pass the placenta and could cause ill effects to the offspring. These might include ill effects similar to those seen in the adult such as reports in 1948 of the stigma of chronic morphine toxicity of newborn infants of mothers addicted to opiates.

There was an awareness of the possible teratogenic effect in drugs not only as a result of studies of aminopterin, but the report in 1958 of masculinization of female infants born to mothers receiving certain progestational agents during pregnancy.[6] There was an appreciation of undeveloped enzyme systems in the fetus of newborns as illustrated by the reports in 1955 of the toxicity of water soluble Vitamin K[7] preparations and in 1959 on the peculiar susceptibility of the newborn to chloramphenicol.[8]

There was increasing realization, too, that the great advances in drug therapy and the development of clinical pharmacology in the intervening years had rendered the 1938 provisions obsolete.

The Thalidomide tragedy added to the concern and contributed to the prompt passage in 1962 of the Kefauver-Harris Amendments and the promulgation in 1963 of new investigational drug regulations. These measures made mandatory the performance of better and more extensive pharmacologic studies, including reproduction studies, before investigational drugs were administered to man. Previous to this time, a new drug could be distributed for clinical trial provided it was clearly labeled for investigational use only, that the investigator signed the statement that he had facilities to test the drug, and that it would be tested under his supervision only, and that the company kept active records of distribution.

Under the new regulations, however, before an investigational drug may be shipped to a clinical investigator, the sponsor, usually a drug manufacturer, is required to submit to the FDA the information that leads him to believe that it is safe to administer the drug to man. This information is submitted as a Notice of Claimed Exemption for an Investigational Drug, commonly known as an IND.

The type of chemical control information and animal studies considered essential before the drug may be used for the first time in man depends to some degree on the nature of the drug and the proposed clinical study or studies. Amongst the more stringent requirements, however, is the provision that reproduction tests, including teratology screening, must be performed before a new drug is administered to a woman capable of becoming pregnant.

Guidelines for the performance of these tests have been prepared by the Food and Drug Administration and are available on request. These are guidelines rather than rigid requirements; modifications may be acceptable to the Administration but should be discussed in advance of initiation.

The requirements for conducting reproduction studies may be waived, if for example, systemic absorption of the drug can be shown to be negligible. Obvious examples of this type might include soft contact lenses and surgical sutures, both of which have been classified as drugs. It might also apply to a non-absorbed preparation taken orally such as radio-opaque contrast medium and to topically applied preparations where absorption under conditions of use can be shown to be negligible. Exceptions might also be made for drugs used in life-threatening conditions for which available therapy is accepted as being unsafe during pregnancy. This might include drugs used in the treatment of cancer. It is ordinarily a requirement that before these drugs are finally approved for marketing, that the reproduction tests be run with a view to comparing their toxicity with that of other available drugs in the same category.

Currently, three types of reproduction studies are required. For the sake of convenience these are referred to as Segment I, Segment II and Segment III, respectively. If desired these three may be run more or less concurrently, and may be run in conjunction with chronic toxicity tests.

Segment I, the conventional reproduction study has a wide scope and is aimed at providing general information on the effects of drugs on fertility in both sexes, the course of gestation, early and late stages of embryonic and fetal development, lactation and postnatal effects. Thus, it provides an overall pilot screening of the effect of the drug on the entire reproductive process including teratogenesis. Young females are treated for about two weeks before mating and treatment with the drug continues until the animals are killed or their offspring are weaned. Males are dosed for 68-80 days before mating. One half the animals are killed at day 13 and the uterine contents are examined for number, distribution and condition of embryos. Additionally, the presence of empty embryonic implantation sites, indicating early embryonic loss, and any other abnormal conditions of the uterus are noted. The surviving females are permitted to go to term and to litter naturally. Observations are made on the duration of pregnancy, litter size, number and condition of dead pups, and gross anomalies of the newborn. On the basis of the results of this study, a decision may be reached to initiate a second litter study or to study the reproductive performance of the surviving offspring.

Segment II is directed primarily at detecting teratogenic effects. The drug is given to the mother only during the period of organogenesis, e.g. days 6-15 for rats and mice, and days 6-18 for rabbits. The comparatively short period of administration is advantageous should the drug in question be an enzyme inducer. Prolonged administration also may be advantageous in that the mode of administration can more easily follow the proposed human use since only short periods of administration will be required.

Segment II offspring are removed by cesarian section one or two days before term and live and dead fetuses, resorption sites and corpora lutea are examined and recorded. Fetuses are weighed and examined for gross anomalies and in the case of rats or mice, one third are then dissected for detection of visceral anomalies and the rest are cleared and stained for skeletal anomalies. In larger animals, such as rabbits, dogs or monkeys, all fetuses should be examined for external, visceral and skeletal anomalies.

Segment III embraces the perinatal and postnatal period. It is designed to study the effect of the drug administered during the last third of pregnancy and the period of lactation. Of concern is the fact that differentiation of central nervous system continues through late pregnancy and after birth and adverse effects may not be readily recognized in the young animal. Behavioral studies in animals are hard to design, execute and interpret. This is an area which needs further study and development.

An additional area of concern with regard to drugs used in pregnancy lies in the possibility of inducing genetic effects. The Food and Drug Administration is becoming increasingly concerned about the possible mutagenic effects of drugs. At present, recognizing the inadequacy of present procedures and their interpretation, screening for mutagenesis is not required. On occasion it has been requested, particularly in the case of drugs chemically related to known mutagens and of highly toxic antineoplastic agents proposed for less serious indications such as psoriasis or rheumatoid arthritis. Recommended tests include the dominant lethal test in mice, *in vivo* cytogenetics, and the host-mediated assay technique to study for effects of metabolites. Multiple generation studies should be performed if mutagenicity tests are positive. Much remains to be done to demonstrate the reproducibility of results from these tests and their relevance to drug use by humans.

Certain general considerations should be mentioned with regard to the conduct of these reproduction studies, especially Segment II. In the first place the current requirement of the Food and Drug Administration is that teratogenicity studies be performed in at least two species of animals. Guidelines have never specified the species to be used, thus permitting the development of new animal models. Studies in mice, rats and rabbits are accepted. Occasionally studies have been requested in monkeys. Every effort should be made to utilize a species known or believed to metabolize the drug in a similar fashion as man.

The route of administration of the drug should be preferably that planned for clinical administration. If the drug is to be administered orally, the animal should be given the drug by stomach tube or capsule whenever possible rather than by incorporation with the diet. If a drug used clinically as a dermal preparation is to be tested for teratogenic potential it may be applied topically under occlusive covering or it can be given orally if absorption can be established by the oral route.

Drug dosage should be at least at two levels. The highest dose should be the maximal tolerated dose, that is the dose just below that which might cause anorexia, sedation or other pharmacologic effects that in themselves may lead to adverse effects on pregnancy. If in the doses used, embryocidal but not the teratogenic effects are seen, dosage would be lowered with a view to determining whether there is a level at which anomalies rather than death may be produced. The use of control groups of animals is essential in view of the incidence of resorptions and malformations in the various species and strains of animals. A positive control is of value in detecting a fluctuation of susceptibility in the animal colony.

The reproduction studies should be performed using an adequate number of animals. It is recommended that at least 20 female mice or rats be used per test group and a minimum for rabbits should be 10 pregnant females. High numbers should be used where practical. Absence of ill effects in comparatively small groups should not lead to complacency. It is for that reason that tests are required to be run at doses considerably higher than those that might be expected to be used clinically.

In the case of preparations that contain two or more active drugs, teratology screening of the preparation is not required if each active ingredient, when tested separately, has been found to be without adverse effects, unless there is evidence of a toxicological or pharmacological interaction between the two drugs. However, if one or more of the ingredients has shown an adverse effect on reproduction when tested individually, additional studies must be carried out on the combination, in view of a possible synergistic or additive effect.

Finally, it is extremely important that reproduction studies like all animal tests, be conducted under optimum conditions for animal care, and by well-trained and conscientious personnel.

The question frequently asked is whether teratology studies performed in countries other than the United States would be acceptable to the Food and Drug Administration. The answer is that provided the qualifications and facilities of the investigator or of the laboratory doing the studies are known to the Administration and considered acceptable, the data will receive the same weight as that generated in the United States, provided, of course, the protocol was compatible with current requirements.

It is generally conceded that the required animal teratology studies, as well as other preclinical studies, serve largely as alerting measures before human studies are undertaken. Such studies, when properly executed, may furnish extremely pertinent and important information with regard to safety in man. However, the practical limitations in numbers of animals used, and the limits of animal models applicable to man, must be taken into account. Should clinical trials reveal toxicity unanticipated on the basis of animal studies, human testing can be halted while more extensive and sophisticated animal studies are performed.

Adverse findings reported during thorough teratologic screening tests must be considered seriously, but do not necessarily preclude the use of the drug in women of childbearing age. Factors that should be taken into consideration by the sponsor of the drug, by the Food and Drug Administration, or by the practicing physician, should include such things as the condition or conditions for which the drug is to be used in man, the dosage required in animals to produce adverse effects, the no-effect dose and any information that may be available concerning possible differences in the metabolism of the drug in man and the animal species in which adverse findings have been observed. On occasion, it may be deemed appropriate to recommend or require screening

201

tests over and beyond those prescribed in the existing guidelines. Thus, if a drug shows adverse effects in common laboratory species such as the rat or rabbit, the sponsor may be advised to perform teratology tests in a subhuman primate species. In other areas of reproduction, if a drug appears to suppress spermatogenesis, additional animal studies may be requested to study the effect in more detail and particularly to establish whether or not the effect is reversible.

When a drug has been approved for marketing by the FDA, the labeling must include appropriate information to guide the physician in its use, including adverse effects; pharmacological and toxicological data; and any other information or precautions including information on its safe use in pregnancy and in children.

Information for use in pregnancy must include any adverse effects noted in pregnant animals and any meaningful information relative to safety in human pregnancy that may have been obtained during the time the drug was under clinical trial. If either or both animal studies or human experience are inadequate, this information must also be stated. In the absence of well-controlled data to indicate safe use of the drug in human pregnancy, the physician must weigh possible therapeutic benefits against possible risks to the mother and to the fetus when administering the drug to pregnant patients or to patients who may become pregnant while taking the drug.

Unfortunately, once a drug is released on the market, no satisfactory method has yet been devised to ensure continuous monitoring of its effects. A step in this direction has been taken recently when an occasional unique drug has been released following minimal human studies consistent with safety for the proposed use, with the understanding that studies will continue post-marketing in a reasonably large group of subjects, the so-called Phase IV studies. It is unlikely, however, that any such Phase IV study would involve sufficient numbers of pregnant women to give adequate information with regard to safety in pregnancy. A commendable step along these lines has been taken by the establishment of an International Registry of Lithium Babies, originated in Denmark by Dr. Schou in cooperation with the American Registry established at the Langley-Porter Neuropsychiatric Institute by Dr. Goldfeld and Dr. Weinstein, and the Canadian Registry established by Dr. Villeneuve in Montreal. These registries collect on a voluntary basis information concerning the outcome of pregnancy in women undergoing Lithium treatment.[9]

The Food and Drug Administration maintains an adverse reaction recording system in which teratogenic effects as well as other adverse effects associated with the drug use are collected and stored in a manner permitting rapid retrieval. Such adverse effects are received from the manufacturer, from physicians and from the public.

Despite more stringent preclinical testing requirements and improved methods of surveillance[10] since the Thalidomide tragedy, no additional drug has been definitely established as a teratogen, although one or two have come under suspicion in this regard. However, there is little room for complacency or for the relaxing of requirements. The incidence of readily recognizable congenital defects at birth remains in the 1-4% range and the vast majority of these are yet of unknown etiology. The serious nature of many birth defects is such that if a drug elicits such effects only in the small segment of the population that may be susceptible, that drug should be considered inacceptable for use during pregnancy if alternate, safer therapy is available. The sample size required to detect small but significant increases in the incidence taxes the scope of present testing methodology. For example, to detect an increase in incidence from 1 per 1,000 to 5 per 1,000 with 90% certainty would require a sample size of 2,795 exposures to the drug at the critical time in pregnancy and a comparable group of non-exposed individuals.

The handful of drugs established to date as teratogens in man were recognized in a large part because the malformations they induce were externally conspicuous. A drug that elicited visceral anomalies only or one that had an embryocidal rather than a teratogenic effect at the therapeutic dose range would be even less readily detected. This would also apply to a drug that elicited an effect that was not manifest until years after birth, such as the apparent relationship between the use of diethylstilbestrol in pregnancy and the development of cancer of the vagina in female offspring at the time of puberty.[11]

The need for the development of improved methodologies for safety evaluation of potentially hazardous chemicals to which man may be exposed led to the establishment in 1971 of the National Center for Toxicological Research at Pine Bluff, Arkansas. This Center, which became operational on May 1, 1972 is administered by the Food and Drug Administration and serves as a national resource shared by the Environmental Protection Agency, other federal agencies, industry and the academic community.

The center will examine the biological effects of pesticides, food additives and therapeutic agents, with particular emphasis on determining the effects of long exposure to low doses of chemicals. The mission of the Center will be accomplished by research studies in 4 core program areas, namely: acute and subacute studies, chronic life-time studies, metabolism studies and teratologic studies. The teratology program will include the evaluation of the teratogenic potential of selected compounds using current techniques. It will also extend to a refinement and improvement of these techniques and the exploration of new approaches to relating data from experimental animals to human safety.

Hopefully, the information will provide more effective regulations pertaining to the safety and effectiveness of new drugs.

REFERENCES

1. E.M.K. Geiling and P.R. Cannon, *J.A.M.A. 111,* 919, 1938.

2. G. Woodard and H.O. Calvery, *Indus. Med. 12,* 55, 1943.

3. Assoc. of Food and Drug Officials of the U. S., *in* Appraisal of the Safety of Chemicals in Food, Drugs and Cosmetics, 1959.

4. J.B. Thiersch, *Am. J. Obstet. Gynec. 63,* 1298, 1952.

5. H.J. Meltzer, *J.A.M.A. 161,* 1253, 1956.

6. M.M. Grumbach, J.R. Ducharme and R. Moloshok, *J. Clin. Endocr. 19,* 1369, 1959.

7. A.C. Allison, *Lancet I,* 669, 1955.

8. J.M. Sutherland, *A.M.A.J. Dis. Child. 97 (6),* 761, 1959.

9. M. Goldfield and M.R. Weinstein, *Amer. J. Psychiat. 127 (7),* 888, 1971.

10. E.B. Hook, D.T. Janerich and I.H. Porter (Eds.), *in* Monitoring, Birth Defects and Environment: The Problem of Surveillance, Academic Press, New York, 1971.

11. A.I. Herbst, H. Ulfelder and D.C. Poskanzer, *N. Engl. J. Med. 284,* 878, 1971.

AN ANALYSIS OF TERATOGENIC TESTING PROCEDURES*

William M. Layton

I am going to discuss three related topics. First, the logical basis for teratogenicity testing. Second, how one might ideally go about designing teratogenicity tests on such a basis. Finally, to consider why some compounds which have been demonstrated to be teratogenic for small laboratory animals do not appear to be so for higher primates including man. I shall make two specific limitations: first, I shall define teratogenic effect as one characterized by malformation resulting from disruption of a normal morphogenetic process. Second, I shall restrict my discussion to the testing of drugs for teratogenicity, although most of what I shall say should apply to other substances as well. I shall not consider in any detail the questions of species to be used or the amount, time or routes of administration of the drugs being tested. This has been very thoroughly covered in several recent reviews.[1,2] Instead, I shall be concerned with the general principles which I feel are useful in the design and interpretation of teratogenicity tests.

THE LOGICAL BASIS OF TERATOGENICITY TESTING

Teratogenicity testing is a special kind of toxicity testing. The rationale of toxicity testing is based on the assumption that man and laboratory animals are similar in their overall reactivity to the particular agent being tested. To the extent that this assumption is true, a test can be said to have predictive value. In teratogenicity testing, however, we must assume that the embryo, placenta and membranes of the two species have similar reactivities. What do these assumptions involve? To find out, it is helpful to dissect the general assumption of similarity into its parts. When we do this, we find that the human patient and the laboratory animal are assumed to be similar in a great many different ways. I should now like to examine these assumptions of similarity, one by one.

---

*This work was supported by N.I.H. Grant ES00697.

WILLIAM M. LAYTON

ASSUMPTIONS OF PHARMACOKINETIC SIMILARITIES

Here we assume similarities in the kinetics of absorption, distribution, metabolism and excretion of the drug being tested. It must be kept in mind that we must consider not only the pharmacokinetics of the drug in the mother, but also the kinetics of transfer of the drug and its metabolites between the mother and the embryo-placental unit* and also the kinetics of the drug in the embryo-placental unit itself. To simplify the situation, I shall first consider the kinetics of the drug in the mother alone. There may be differences not only between the human patient and the laboratory animal but also between the pregnant and non-pregnant human patient. This can be due to pregnancy-associated changes in drug distribution caused by changes in compartment size and changes in hormone activity which may alter rates of drug metabolism. Also, drug metabolism may be altered by interaction with other drugs.[3,4] This is particularly important since it is unusual for a patient to be taking only a single drug.

Next are the kinetics of exchange of drug metabolite between mother and embryo. In the human patient, this exchange occurs chiefly at the chorio-allantoic placenta. However, in laboratory rodents and the rabbit, two placentas are functional during organ formation. These are the yolk sac (choriovitelline) placenta and the chorioallantoic placenta. These two organs are probably quite different in their exchange characteristics and, during the time of organ formation, change in their relative importance to the embryo. In early embryogenesis, the yolk sac placenta is the principal organ of exchange but, later, the chorioallantoic placenta predominates. Also, both placentas show progressive morphological changes during pregnancy, so that placental function is probably quite different in early and late pregnancy. In the human subject, it is uncertain whether or not the yolk sac functions as an organ of maternal-embryonic exchange in early pregnancy.[5] Transfer across the placenta probably takes place by the following mechanisms:[6] diffusion, facilitated diffusion, active transport, pinocytosis, and through membrane discontinuities.

Surprisingly little is known about the transfer functions of the early placenta in the human patient. There are a number of papers in the literature dealing with placental transfer at or around the time of birth[6-11] in both the human patient and experimental animal. However, it is doubtful if such studies are of much value in the prediction of placental transfer characteristics

---

*It is important to use the term "embryo-placental unit" rather than "feto-placental unit" to emphasize that it is the embryo, not the fetus, that is susceptible to teratogenic action.

during early development when organs are being formed.

Next, I should like to consider the kinetics of a drug in the embryo-placental unit. Here we know very little and can only speculate about orders of complexity. In the most simple situation, there might only be three effective compartments (intracellular, interstitial and vascular) for drug (or metabolite) distribution. On the other hand, there may be many more compartments. The interstitial and intracellular compartments of the placenta may be functionally separate from those of the embryo. Also, the amniotic cavity and yolk sac might each be functionally separate from those of the embryo. Whatever the situation, it is quite possible for a drug or its metabolites to be selectively concentrated in or excluded from one of these compartments.

From all of the above considerations, it is not reasonable to assume, without specific evidence, that the pregnant human patient and the pregnant laboratory animal are similar with respect to the pharmacokinetics of any particular drug: there are simply too many variables involved.

ASSUMPTIONS OF SIMILARITIES IN BIOTRANSFORMATION IN MAN AND EXPERIMENTAL ANIMALS

It is well known that a toxic drug may be transformed to a nontoxic metabolite or that the reverse may take place. Also, metabolic patterns may be changed by drug interaction or altered by physiological states or disease. Here again are possible differences not only between the laboratory animal and human patient but between pregnant and non-pregnant human patient. In considerations of similarities and differences, the many different possible sites for biotransformation must be kept in mind. Besides biotransformation by the mother, the placenta and embryo are also possible sites. While the placenta has been known for some time as a site for the biotransformation of steroid hormones,[12–14] recent work has shown that it is also capable of biotransformation of drugs.[15–17] It is also possible that the embryo itself is active in biotransformation. Although direct evidence about this is not available, biotransformation of several organic compounds by the early fetus has been demonstrated.[16] Several recent studies have shown that a great many different enzymes appear very early in embryogenesis[18,19] and, although the enzymes detected are not involved (as far as I know) in the biotransformation of drugs, it seems reasonable to assume that such enzymes occur in the early embryo. Again, we see that we cannot assume, without further evidence, that man and laboratory animal are similar with respect to the way they metabolize a particular drug.

WILLIAM M. LAYTON

ASSUMPTIONS OF SIMILARITIES IN THE REACTIVITIES OF THE EMBRYOS OF MAN AND EXPERIMENTAL ANIMALS

In consideration of the embryonic reactivity to teratogens, it must be kept in mind that while the embryo is the ultimate site of teratogenic action, the primary site may be elsewhere. Thus, the embryo may not react directly to the drug (or metabolite) itself, but rather secondarily to drug induced changes in the mother, placenta or embryonic membranes. This distinction is important since it appears that among different species there is a greater similarity in the way that an embryo reacts to direct drug effects than to indirect ones. This is probably because a smaller number of variables are involved when a drug acts directly on the embryo. As a first approximation, we may assume that the reactivity of embryonic morphogenetic processes to direct action of a teratogen are similar from one mammalian species to another and that this similarity is greatest at the cellular level, less so at the tissue level and least at the level of the morphogenesis of the entire embryo. The morphogenetic processes on a cellular level which are quite similar from species to species include: cell division, changes in cell shape, cell migration, selective cell sorting and aggregation, and normal ("programmed") cell death. Substances which act at this level may be expected to show inter-specific similarities. For instance, substances like nitrogen mustard which interfere with cell division will do so to the cells of most species. Similarly, substances which interfere with the formation of microtubules and micro-filaments, and thus affect cell shape, may be expected to be active over a wide range of species. Colchicine and cytochalasin B are two such substances.

On the other hand, at the level of complexity of organ formation, a number of interdependent sequential steps of cell and tissue morphogenesis are involved and it is unlikely that all of these steps will be similar in their reactivities to teratogens. It is at this level that species (or even strains) often show a predilection for specific kinds of malformations. This is probably due to a particular weak link in a long and complex chain of morphogenetic processes. Thus, we see that while we are reasonably safe in assuming similarities in embryonic reactivities at the cellular level, similarities at higher levels of complexity are less likely. However, taken as a whole, the interspecific variability of embryonic reactivity is not as great as the variability of pharmacokinetics or biotransformation.

CONSEQUENCES OF INTERSPECIFIC DIFFERENCES IN PHARMACO-KINETICS, BIOTRANSFORMATION OR EMBRYONIC REACTIVITY

I have tried to demonstrate the very large number of variables involved in

208

the production of malformations in any one species by a particular drug. Since it is unlikely that two species would be alike in so many different ways, it follows that it is unlikely that they will show the same overall reactivity to a teratogenic agent. As a matter of fact, two inbred strains of the same species may react quite differently to a teratogen. This has been shown, for instance, by Dr. Fraser and his colleagues in their work with cortisone-induced cleft palate in mice.[20] If we fail to demonstrate carry-over of results within members of the same species, it seems unreasonable to expect it between members of different species. However, this is exactly what we do when we perform teratogenicity tests as they are usually designed. In what I shall call a one-stage test, a drug is given to several species of pregnant animals and the offspring are examined for malformations. There are usually no appropriate data on pharmacokinetics or biotransformation which would aid in the selection of an appropriate species or a sensible route of administration, or even the suitable compound to use (the parent drug or a metabolite). Some effort is made to get around these difficulties by using several species and, sometimes, with luck, this approach may work. It is little wonder that there is such poor correlation between the results of one-stage animal tests and the ultimate findings in human patients.

I would like to suggest that in order to increase the predictive value of an animal test, it should be done as a series of experiments. The design of each experiment should depend on the findings of earlier ones. How might such a test be conducted? First, studies of pharmacokinetics and biotransformation should be done in laboratory animals and then in non-pregnant human subjects. The next step might be to see if the drug or metabolite crossed the placenta and, if so, in what form. Here, a non-human primate might be a suitable test animal. In this case, we need only assume that the monkey is similar to man in the way the placenta functions in biotransformation and transfer, not in its overall reactivity to a teratogen. A test of this sort should not require many monkeys. If the material is transferred, a more uniform and available experimental animal can be sought that has similar placental transfer characteristics with respect to the drug being tested. The teratogenicity test would then be done in this animal. While we would still have to make assumptions about similarities in the reactivity of the embryo-placental unit, the overall predictive value of the test would be much greater for having been done in sequential steps.

SOME EXAMPLES OF THE IMPORTANCE OF PHARMACOKINETICS AND BIOTRANSFORMATION

At this point, I should like to illustrate what I have said with several examples of varying degrees of complexity. First, I should like to consider an antimitotic agent such as nitrogen mustard. We have already seen that it should be expected to be teratogenic if it can reach the embryo. In this case it would be sufficient to demonstrate that the drug or a metabolite with similar activity reached the embryo in adequate amounts. Further testing would be unnecessary. Similarly, a drug with demonstrated androgenic activity which can be shown to reach the embryo will quite probably produce masculinization of the female human embryo if given at sufficient dosage at the proper time in pregnancy. In both of these cases, the problems are of pharmacokinetics and biotransformation, not of embryonic reactivity.

There are yet other examples which illustrate the importance of knowing something about the pharmacokinetics and biotransformation of a drug. It has been found that cyclopia can be produced in sheep and other ruminants by ingestion of the weed *Veratrum californicum*.[21] Studies have demonstrated that this malformation is induced by any of three alkaloids of closely related structure.[22] One of these alkaloids, appropriately named cyclopamine, was given to rabbits and found not to be teratogenic.[23] However, it was found that this species-related difference in reactivity was due to the much higher gastric acidity of the rabbit when compared to the ruminant. Under conditions of low pH, cyclopamine was transformed to veratramine, an inactive compound. When cyclopamine was administered to rabbits along with sufficient alkali, it was teratogenic and, in fact, produced cyclopia.

Another pertinent study is that of Kimmel, Wilson and Schumacher[24] on aspirin. They showed that aspirin is a teratogen in the rat and that in this species, the aspirin is transformed to salicylic acid which is transferred across the placenta and acts directly on the embryo as a teratogen. They then cited evidence that the biotransformation of aspirin is the same in the human subject as in the rat and, furthermore, that it can cross the human placenta. From this, they conclude that the teratogenic risk of aspirin for the human cannot be discounted. They also point out that the simultaneous administration of benzoic acid (a commonly used food preservative) with aspirin results in higher and more prolonged salicylate levels and that this combination would increase the teratogenicity of the aspirin. Unfortunately, the only data that they could find in the literature about salicylate crossing the human placenta was a report of a full term pregnancy in which a very large quantity of aspirin had been ingested with suicidal intent.[25] Here it would be of interest to learn whether a more modest dose might result in significant salicylate levels in the early embryo. One way to learn more about this would

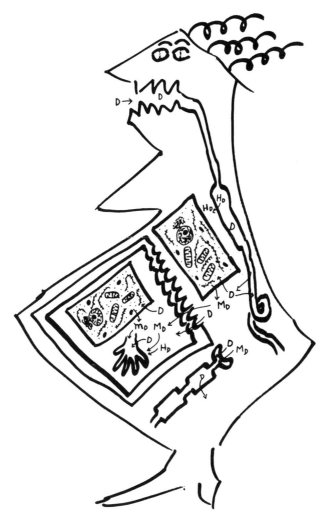

Figure 1. Here we can see the complexity of the pharmacokinetics and biotransformation of a drug (D) in a pregnant patient. It may be hydrolyzed in the stomach (H_D); it may be metabolized, for instance by a liver cell (note mitochondria and endoplasmic reticulum) to a metabolite (M_D). The drug or metabolite may be transferred across the placenta to the embryo, where it may be metabolized (note mitochondria, etc.) and the drug or metabolite may then produce malformations. The drug or its metabolite may be excreted by the kidney (note nephron) before or after (or without) being transferred to the embryo.

be to measure salicylate levels of maternal plasma and embryonic tissue in patients undergoing therapeutic abortion early in pregnancy. A similar study was actually done by Uno.[26] He measured the concentration of thiopental in the maternal blood and its concentration, as well as those of metabolites, in the tissues of the abortus. He found that although the maternal plasma concentration of thiopental was higher than that of the embryo, the embryo contained a higher concentration of pentobarbital, a metabolite. Since he was working with embryos (not fetuses) and since he showed comparable results in experiments done with mice, and since pentobarbital cannot be demonstrated to be teratogenic for mice, one can say, with some assurance, that neither thiopental nor pentobarbital constitute a teratogenic risk for the human patient.

AGENTS PROVEN TO BE TERATOGENIC FOR LABORATORY ANIMALS AND WHICH DO NOT APPEAR TO BE TERATOGENIC FOR MAN

There are a number of agents which have been reported to cause malformations in laboratory animals, but not in man. Obviously, if something is found to be teratogenic in animals, it is not likely to be given to human subjects. If such human "trials" occur (and they are rare) they are frequently accidental and the data often unreliable. However, there are instances in which large human populations containing many women in early pregnancy have been exposed to agents prior to the accumulation of data which proved these agents to be teratogenic for laboratory animals. The agents that come immediately to mind are: aspirin (mentioned above), vitamin A deficiency,[27] caffeine,[28,29] and acetazolamide,[30] and I am sure that there are others. If we are investigating the predictive value of teratogenicity tests, we should try to explain these failures. There are many possible explanations. It is possible that human malformations are produced but the causal relationship is not recognized. This is unlikely, however, since epidemiological surveillance techniques are in use which should detect such a relationship, especially since individual teratogens tend to cause reproducible spectra of malformations in any one species. Since this has been dealt with in a previous conference here[31] and at this conference, I shall not discuss it further. Other possible explanations seem much more likely. The dose-response curve may be quite steep and the usual human dose may simply not be high enough. There may be associated differences in pharmacokinetics or biotransformation.

There is also some evidence that small laboratory animals may be more susceptible to teratogens than are the higher primates. In a recent paper, Wilson[32] compared the teratogenicity of nine selected compounds in the rat and monkey. He found that a smaller dose was necessary for an embryopathic effect in the rat and that such an effect was more likely to result in malformation in the rat and death of the embryo in the monkey. I would like to suggest that this increased susceptibility of the rat to teratogens might be associated with a large reproductive potential and that the selective advantage of having many large litters (a capacity the rat shares with many other small mammals) may have been gained at the expense of an increased susceptibility to environmental teratogens. In this regard, the yolk sac placenta, an embryonic adaptation which allows a shorter period of gestation, is itself the specific target of at least one teratogen, trypan blue. Since many of the adaptations to increase the reproductive potential probably involve modifications of the placenta and membranes, it is quite likely that a great deal of species-associated variation in sensitivity to teratogens is due to such modifications. Since the placenta and embryonic membranes are important in maintaining the proper microenvironment for the developing embryo, interference with this homeostatic function would most probably be teratogenic. I would like to discuss the possible mechanism of teratogenicity because its importance may not be generally appreciated and also because I have been doing some work in this field. First, I should like to point out that the mammalian embryo lives in an environment the composition of which is more closely regulated than is the internal environment of the mother. This has been particularly well shown for electrolyte concentration.[33-35] Concentrations of electrolytes in maternal plasma can be varied through a wide range without significantly changing the ion concentrations of the embryo. This is similar in many ways to the situation in the central nervous system where the composition of the cerebrospinal fluid has been found to be very closely regulated in the face of wide fluctuations of plasma composition.[36]

One of the agents studied by Wilson and demonstrated to be a teratogen in rats and not in monkeys was the carbonic anhydrase inhibitor, acetazolamide. This drug was at one time widely used as a diuretic agent, often in early pregnancy. In spite of this, there is no evidence that acetazolamide has ever produced human malformations although it has been demonstrated to be a teratogen in mice and hamsters as well as rats.[30,37] The malformations produced are highly specific in their structure and localization. In rats and mice it involves the postaxial part of the right fore-limb, usually consisting of an ectrodactyly. In hamsters either fore-limb may be involved (the malformation is still postaxial) and occasionally the left hind-limb is also malformed. The hind foot deformities are not seen in the rat or mouse and, with rare exceptions, the malformations described above are the only ones produced.

This is in contrast to most other teratogens which usually produce a wide variety of deformities. The mechanism of action appears to involve carbonic anhydrase inhibition since similar malformations can be produced by other potent carbonic anhydrase inhibitors with quite different chemical structures.[38-40] However, at the time of gestation that these enzyme inhibitors act, there is no demonstrable carbonic anhydrase in the embryo,[40] so that the site of action must be extraembryonic, either in the mother or in the embryoplacental unit. Scott[41] has shown that a very small amount of acetazolamide injected directly into a single implantation site of the rat produced malformations of the embryo at that location alone. We have confirmed this finding in hamsters.[42] This means that acetazolamide probably acts on either the chorioallantoic or choriovitelline (yolk sac) placenta. Maren and Ellison[35] have presented evidence that there is ion imbalance, particularly of potassium in both the mother and embryo. It appears, then, that the normal homeostatic mechanism of the embryo has been disrupted by inhibition of placental carbonic anhydrase and the resulting ion imbalance is responsible for the malformations. Grabowski[43] showed that ionic or fluid imbalance could cause malformations in the chick embryo and suggested that this might also be teratogenic for mammals. It is tempting to speculate that it is the yolk sac placenta that is involved, since this would give an explanation for the lack of teratogenicity of acetazolamide for higher primates.

Finally, I should like to point out that acetazolamide affords a unique opportunity to learn about the mechanism of action of a teratogen. There are no problems involving pharmacokinetics or biotransformation, since in rats (and probably other rodents) this drug is widely distributed, reaches the embryo in concentrations similar to those found in maternal tissues and it is not metabolized. Its chief (and probably only) activity is the inhibition of carbonic anhydrase, an enzyme of unusually wide distribution (it is present in all vertebrates, many invertebrates and even some plants). The malformations it produces are very specific and it causes no other lasting deleterious effects on the embryo.

CONCLUSION

I have tried to emphasize the importance of a rational approach to teratogenicity testing. This involves learning first about the pharmacokinetics and biotransformation of a drug and then using these data to test the drug in an appropriate species using an appropriate route of administration. To illustrate the complexities of pharmacokinetics and biotransformation, I refer you to Figure 1. I have also examined the correlation between the results of animal tests and the ultimate findings in human patients and pointed out some possible reasons for the rather poor showing. I am firmly convinced that we can give animal tests greater predictive value if we follow a sequential experimental design rather than sticking blindly to the one state teratogenicity test which is now usually considered adequate.

REFERENCES

1. R.L. Cahen, *Clin. Pharmacol. Ther. 5,* 480, 1964.

2. H. Tuchmann-Duplessis, *Teratology 5,* 271, 1972.

3. J.E. Gibson and B.A. Becker, *Teratology 1,* 393, 1968.

4. J.E. Gibson and B.A. Becker, *J. Pharmacol. Exp. Therap. 177,* 256, 1971.

5. E.W. Dempsey, *in* Methods for Teratological Studies in Animals and Man, Nishimura, Miller and Yasuda (Eds.), Igaku Shoin, Tokyo, p. 155, 1969.

6. J. Asling and E.C. Way, *in* Fundamentals of Drug Metabolism and Drug Disposition, LaDu, Mandel and Way (Eds.), Williams & Wilkins, Baltimore, p. 88, 1972.

7. C.A. Villee, *Ann. N.Y. Acad. Sci. 123,* 237, 1965.

8. M.G. Horning, C.D. Waterbury, E.C. Horning and R.M. Hill, *in* The Feto-placental Unit, Excerpta Medica, Amsterdam, 1969.

9. R.L. Schultz, *Obstet. Gynec. Survey 25,* 979, 1970.

10. M.A. Heyman, *Fed. Proc. 31,* 44, 1972.

11. L.D. Longo, *in* Pathology of Gestation, N. Assali (Ed.), Academic Press, New York, p. 1, 1972.

12. B. Brinck-Johnsen and K. Benirschke, *in* Endocrine Pathology, J. Bloodworth (Ed.), Williams & Wilkins, Baltimore, 1968.

13. H.H. Simmer, *in* Pathology of Gestation, N. Assali (Ed.),Vol. 1, Ch. 5, Academic Press, New York 1972.

14. H.H. Simmer, *in* Pathophysiology of Gestation, N. Assali and C.R. Brinckman (Eds.), Vol. 1, Academic Press, New York, 1972.

15. A.J. Szabo and R.D. Grimbaldi, *Adv. Metab. Dis. 4,* 185, 1970.

16. O. Pelkonen, P. Arvela and N.T. Körki, *Acta Pharmacol. Toxicol. 30,* 395, 1971.

17. M.R. Juchau, *Fed. Proc. 31,* 48, 1972.

18. E.M. Johnson, K. Takano and H. Nishimura, *Teratology, 5,* 89, 1972.

19. C.J. Masters and R.S. Holmes, *Biol. Rev. 47,* 309, 1972.

20. F.C. Fraser, *in* Methods for Teratological Studies in Animals and Man, Nishimura, Miller and Yasuda (Eds.), Igaku Shoin, Tokyo, p. 115, 1969.

21. W. Binns, L.F. James, J.L. Schube and G. Everett, *Am. J. Vet. Res. 24,* 1164, 1963.

22. R.F. Keeler, *Teratology 3,* 175, 1970.

23. R.F. Keeler and W. Binns, *Teratology 1,* 5, 1968.

24. C.A. Kimmel, J.G. Wilson and H. Schumacher, *Teratology 4,* 15, 1971.

25. A.V. Jackson, *J. Path. Bact. 60,* 587, 1948.

26. T. Uno, *in* Methods for Teratological Studies in Animals and Man, Nishimura, Miller and Yasuda (Eds.), Igaku Shoin, Tokyo, p. 121, 1969.

27. J. Warkany, *in* Congenital Malformations, Notes and Comments, Yearbook Publishers, Chicago, p. 129, 1971.

28. H. Nishimura and K. Nakai, *Proc.Soc. exp. Biol Med. 104,* 140, 1960.

29. M. Bertrand, E. Schwan, A. Frandon and J. Alary, *Comp. Rend. Soc. Biol. 159,* 2199, 1965.

30. W.M. Layton and D.W. Hallesy, *Science 149,* 306, 1965.

31. E.B. Hook, D.T. Janerich and I.H. Porter (Eds.), *in* Monitoring, Birth Defects and Environment, Academic Press, New York, 1971.

32. J.G. Wilson, *Fed. Proc. 30,* 104, 1971.

33. E.L. Stewart and E.G. Welt, *Amer. J. Physiol. 200,* 824, 1961.

34. A.C. Ellison and T.H. Maren, *Johns Hopkins Med. J. 130,* 105, 1972.

35. T.H. Maren and A.C. Ellison, *Johns Hopkins Med. J. 130,* 87, 1972.

36. H. Cserr, *Physiol. Rev. 51,* 272, 1971.

38. J.G. Wilson, T.H. Maren and K. Takano, *Abst. Terat. Soc. 6,* 30, 1966.

39. D.W. Hallesy and W.M. Layton, *Proc. Soc. Exp. Biol. Med. 126,* 6, 1967.

40. J.G. Wilson, T.H. Maren, K. Takano and A. Ellison, *Teratology 1,* 51, 1968.

41. W.J. Scott, *Teratology 3,* 261, 1970.

42. A.J. Storch and W.M. Layton, Jr., *Teratology,* (in press), 1973.

43. C.T. Grabowski, *Science 142,* 1064, 1963.

EXPERIMENTAL VIRUS-INDUCED CONGENITAL DEFECTS:
THE PATHOGENESIS OF FETAL HOG CHOLERA INFECTIONS*

Kenneth P. Johnson
David P. Byington

Viruses, at least rubella and human cytomegalovirus, are among the best defined environmental causes of sporadic human birth defects. Nevertheless, the vast majority of fetal malformations, which complicate between 2% and 4% of live human births,[1] have no discernible cause. Recently, several common congenital malformations of the human central nervous system (CNS) have been duplicated in virus-infected domestic and experimental animals. We wish to outline some of these studies briefly, and then describe in more detail the mechanisms by which live vaccine strains of Hog Cholera Virus (HCV) produce several significant defects in fetal swine.

Several years ago, Johnson and Johnson[2] reported the production of aqueductal stenosis and hydrocephalus as delayed sequela of acute infections of newborn hamsters with mumps, influenza and para-influenza I viruses. In these studies, the intracerebrally inoculated viruses replicated primarily in ependymal cells rapidly denuding the ventricular surface. Weeks or months later, when all histologic evidence of the preceding infection had disappeared, progressive, often fatal, hydrocephalus became apparent. The degree of glial reaction observed in the periaqueductal area was a function of age,[3] for in the newborn animal no secondary glial reaction developed, thus duplicating the appearance of idiopathic, congenital aqueductal forking or atresia noted in man. When older rodents were infected with influenza A virus, aqueductal narrowing also occurred, but was accompanied by an increase in periaqueductal glial fibers, similar to aqueductal gliosis often noted in human hydrocephalus, and thought to be secondary to some preceding inflammatory condition. Experimental infections of rodents with reo I virus[4] and Ross River arboviruses[5] have also led to aqueductal stenosis and hydrocephalus. Reo I

---

*This work was supported by PHS grant NS-08808 and a grant from the National Foundation (North East Ohio Chapter).

virus was shown to cross the placenta and infect fetal ependymal cells, thus furthering the possible analogy with congenital hydrocephalus in man.

Mumps virus is the most common viral agent known to invade the human CNS.[6] Recently, mumps encephalitis has been established as a cause of delayed aqueductal stenosis in children.[7] However, no evidence exists at present directly linking intra-uterine mumps infections with congenital hydrocephalus in man.

Early chick embryos, infected with influenza A virus, often develop focal non-closure and flexion abnormalities of the neural tube. These phenomena occur rapidly, always leading to the death of the embryo; nevertheless, they suggest early events which may be occurring in the development of spina bifida. These neural tube abnormalities have been shown to be an indirect effect of influenza infection, which is limited to extra-neural cells[8] indicating that the areas of virus replication in the fetus may differ from the location of the ultimate structural abnormality noted in an older malformed fetus or infant.

Recently, Osborn et al.[9] have described the production of hydranencephaly and porencephalic cysts in sheep fetuses inoculated directly with live virus vaccine strains of Blue Tongue virus (BTV). Immunofluorescent studies showed that virus replicated primarily in dividing and migrating subependymal cells and primitive neurons, causing acute cellular destruction, accompanied by an active, but brief inflammatory response. When the infection was initiated on the 50th day of the 150 day ovine gestational period, cells of the subependymal plate were the primary viral target and typical hydranencephaly was later found at birth. If, however, the infection was begun on day 75 of gestation, migrating primitive cerebral cortical neurons and glia were infected in a focal pattern, resulting in multiple porencephalic cysts in the cerebral hemispheres at term. Infection begun on day 100, failed to produce CNS defects. In these studies, cerebellar lesions were not noted, indicating a remarkable variation in the susceptibility of primitive CNS cells for BTV infection.

Hog Cholera Virus

Several years ago, we began a search for a teratogenic virus which could be studied in its natural host, hoping to use it to uncover new mechanisms of fetal infection and malformation, which might not be operative in more contrived experiments in which a human virus was adapted to infect an experimental animal host. It was known that infection with wild strains of HCV, usually manifest by severe enteritis and encephalitis in adult swine, was not usually associated with fetal malformation; perhaps, because the maternal clinical disease was so severe that it produced abortion of the pregnancy.

220

clinical disease was so severe that it porduced abortion of the pregnancy. However, live vaccine strains of HCV, which normally produce little or no clinical disease in the pregnant sow, were teratogenic to varying degrees.[10]

Hog Cholera Virus is an enveloped RNA virus of the Toga virus group to which, interestingly, human rubella virus also belongs. A vaccine strain of HCV which had been attenuated by repeated passages in rabbits, and then in swine, and was known to produce fetal malformations in the field, was used in these studies.

Sows were arbitrarily inoculated subcutaneously on the 30th day of their 114 day gestational period. The only clinical response to infection was a brief period of fever and anorexia for 3 to 5 days. However, between 7 and 18 days after inoculation, approximately 1/3 of the animals spontaneously aborted the pregnancy, indicating that the virus did produce fetal loss, probably by a direct intra-uterine invasion, rather than as an indirect consequence of grave maternal disease. All sows developed serum antibodies to HCV. Virus could not be isolated from any maternal tissue 20 days after inoculation; therefore, the adult pig could limit and terminate the infection.

Sows were sacrificed at 50, 75, 100 and 114 days of gestation for assessment of fetal malformations and collection of tissues. Studies on collected tissues included: assay of virus content, fluorescent antibody staining to determine the cellular localization of viral antigen, evaluation of the serological response, and histological examination for pathological change.

When the fetuses were collected at term, a variety of defects, some of which could be called lesions and others malformations, were apparent. Multiple skin, kidney and spleen petechiae, a hallmark of congenital and postnatal HCV infections, were present. Massive ascites (Fig. 1) associated with a hobnail-like nodularity of the liver, was common and seemed to increase in severity throughout the last half of pregnancy. In approximately 1/3 of term fetuses, a profound hypogenesis of the lungs was observed, even though chest wall, heart and great vessels appeared normal. Rarely, bony malformation of one or both forelimbs, similar to arthrogryposis multiplex congenita, was seen in term fetuses.

All brains from infected fetuses, when examined at term, were abnormal. In many, moderate microcephaly was present, the cerebral hemispheres weighing approximately 70% of control hemispheres. In many brains, the cerebral gyrus pattern was simplified. The cerebellum was markedly hypoplastic in every infected fetus (Fig. 2). This malformation was evident by the 75th day of gestation and became more apparent as the fetus grew. Microscopic study showed that myelin development was markedly retarded in each infected brain at term. Tissue culture and fluorescent antibody studies suggested that the hypomyelinogenesis was secondary to persistent infection of

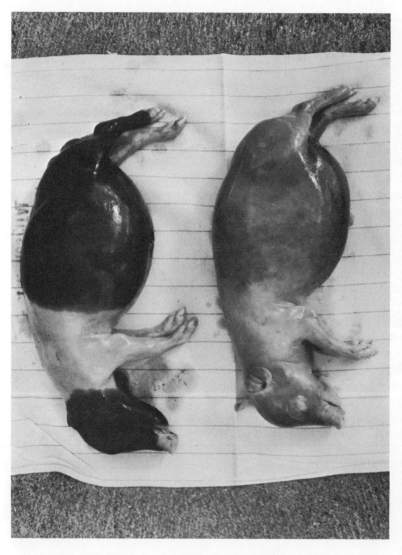

Figure 1. Two fetal swine, both with massive ascites, collected on the 100th day of gestation. The sow had received a live vaccine strain of Hog Cholera Virus subcutaneously on the 30th day of the 114 day porcine gestational period.

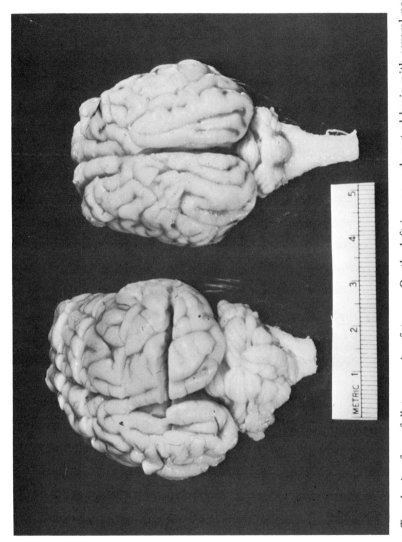

Figure 2. Two brains from full term swine fetuses. On the left is a normal control brain with several postmortem incisions made to improve fixation. On the right is the brain of a fetus removed from a sow that had been inoculated subcutaneously with a live Hog Cholera vaccine virus on the 30th day of gestation. Note the smaller size and the severe cerebellar hypoplasia.

oligodendroglia.

This collection of visceral and CNS abnormalities developed in the course of continued infection, for each fetus developed a persistent viremia soon after inoculation of the sow, and all had virus in the CNS as well, at birth. Although virus was cultured and could be demonstrated in the CNS germinal tissues by fluorescent microscopy, nevertheless, no inflammatory response, no inclusion bearing cells and no unusual cell necrosis was apparent. To date, we have also failed to demonstrate a humeral immune response in fetal blood. These studies strongly suggest that HCV invades, then remains in selected populations of cells in some fetal organs. Once established, it inhibits cell division and maturation, thus causing the observed congenital defects. Focal infection of vascular endothelial cells also may lead to the petechiae noted. The infection is obviously damaging to the fetus; nevertheless, the usual immunological response is either inhibited by the virus or the host fails to recognize it as a foreign antigen.

Discussion

The studies cited in this paper illustrate a variety of experimental virus induced fetal malformations which have counterparts in human fetal pathology. Spina bifida, hydrocephalus, hydraencaphaly, porencephalic cysts, microcephaly and cerebellar hypoplasia are significant malformations in human teratology, yet the cause for most of them is unknown. Many of the experimental lesions bear no stigmata of an infectious process at birth, even though the malformed organs may continue to harbor and shed virus. Thus, histological criteria alone, as a means of ruling out a viral etiology for a human malformation, must be changed or disregarded. More importantly, new virologic and immunologic methods must be employed in an attempt to isolate unique teratogenic agents from the malformed human fetus.

The mechanisms by which viruses induce malformations are extremely varied. The lesions may be the result of rapid destruction of a selected population of cells, such as the attack on migratory telencephalic cells in BTV infections. This process can only occur if the infection is initiated at a specific time. An alternative mechanism is the persistent, but non-cytopathic, infection of CNS germinal cells noted in HCV fetal infections where the virus appears to inhibit, relatively, the division, maturation and migration of various CNS cells. The virus may even produce CNS malformation indirectly by its malignant influence on neighboring extraneural cell groups as in influenza A infections of chick embryos.

Finally, these studies demonstrate that two domestic animal viruses (BTV of sheep and HCV of swine) retain or perhaps develop a teratogenic potential when attenuated for use as live virus vaccines. A similar course of events could occur in human medicine as increasing numbers of live viral agents are being attenuated and employed as vaccines. Viral attenuation prior to deliberate human exposure, may pose a new health threat to developing fetuses, even though the vaccine serves as a defense againse postnatal disease.

REFERENCES

1. L.W. Catalano, Jr. and J.L. Sever, *Ann. Rev. Microbio.* 25, 255, 1971.

2. R.T. Johnson and K.P. Johnson, *Exp. Mol. Path. 10,* 68, 1969.

3. K.P. Johnson and R.T. Johnson, *Am. J. Path. 67,* 511, 1972.

4. G. Margolis and L. Kilham, *Lab. Invest. 21,* 189, 1969.

5. F.A. Murphy, C.A. Mims, I.D. Marshall *et al., Am. Soc. Microbio. 239,* 1972.

6. H.O. Bang and J. Bang, *Acta Med. Scand. 113,* 487, 1943.

7. G.D. Timmons and K.P. Johnson, *N. Eng. J. Med. 283,* 1505, 1970.

8. K.P. Johnson, R. Klasnja and R.T. Johnson, *J. Neuropath. Exp. Neurol. 30,* 68, 1971.

9. B.I. Osborn, R.T. Johnson, A.M. Silverstein *et al., Lab. Invest. 25,* 197, 206, 1971.

10. J.L. Emerson and A.L. Delez, *J.A.M.A. 147,* 47, 1965.

DISCUSSION

DR. HOOK: Dr. Layton, I agree with you entirely in hoping that we can obtain some rational basis for predicting the teratogenicity of drugs and other environmental agents in humans but the problem, as I see it, is that we are far away from being able to establish the pathways by which we could predict the teratogenic effects of any compound.

How plausible would it be to rely exclusively on primate testing? To my knowledge, there are no compounds which are teratogenic in lower organisms and in man but not teratogenic in primates. The only possible exception to this is amethopterin but I think that there is evidence that amethopterin is at least an abortifacient in primates. In man, the effect of amethopterin was primarily fetal wastage and the teratogenic effect was apparent only in those few fetuses that survived the entire period of gestation.

DR. LAYTON: I didn't mean that all testing should be done in primates. As a matter of fact, we can't even use humans for testing because there is considerable heterogeneity in humans. We should really understand what the process is because, as an example, glucose-6-phosphate dehydrogenase deficiency, if it is tested for with a hemolytic drug in the wrong part of the world, we miss that kind of toxicity. What I really meant was that I think that for measuring transfer, one or two primates might be all right.

But, to get back to my original point, I admit it was rather dreamy. I've been involved in tests done in the usual way when the pharmacologists have said: "We just found out that this stuff is completely metabolized." And, so we do the entire test again with a metabolite. Once we did that three times and active compounds kept turning up. As I said, I am really talking about an ideal aim. In fact, I don't think it's wise to start teratogenicity testing before we have some information on pharmacokinetics, biotransformation, etc.

DR. NEWCOMBE: Suppose we were to require that the first hundred thousand prescriptions of a new drug be issued only on the condition that the person should identify himself fully for the purposes of follow-up, that the pharmacist be paid, say 50 cents for collecting this on a standard form and forwarding it to a central agency. Now, the object would be to facilitate studies and the simplest way is to pick out the abnormal children born in the next twelve months. There are, of course, lots of other studies that could be done. What are the administrative, political and other objections to something like this?

DR. KELSEY: In Europe, when the patient picks up the prescription, various factors, such as age, sex, etc., are recorded.

DR. NEWCOMBE: The pharmacist, however, should have a standard form and if you want details, these could also be recorded. Such factors as surname, present address, date of birth, etc., could easily be included on such a form.

DR. KELSEY: If I'm not mistaken, they have done surveys of this type in part of the British Isles where the prescription is part of the health service and, as I recall, one of the difficulties encountered was that the mother's name changed between the time she got the prescription and the time she had a child.

LEON GOLBERG (Albany Medical College, Albany, New York): Equally important as teratology testing are interpretations of the data. Those of us involved are constantly reminded of the importance of this and I'd like to give you two examples to show you the kind of thing we're up against. Let us first take the case of FD and C Red No. 2 where we know that azo dyes of this sort are metabolized by the bacteria in the intestine which obviously have a limited capacity to break these compounds down. Now in the test carried out by FDA, massive doses, as high as 300 mg/kg, were given in a single treatment, that is, by gavage, whereas of course, the ordinary method of ingestion is in food. At a maximum level of 60 ppm and then only in some foods, no toxicity was observed. Now, the Committee appointed by the National Academy of Sciences, of which I was a member, decided that before these results could be interpreted, we needed to know more about metabolism under these test conditions and we needed also to have a clear understanding of what the metabolites, which are known to be produced in man, do in the experimental animal. Now this attitude was labeled by the consumer advocates as white-washing and the Committee as a whole and the National Academy of Sciences were subjected to the usual processes of denigration and insult by the . consumer advocates. We need to have some public statement of the principles which have been set out this morning by Dr. Layton.

Let me just give you another example: in the case of phthalates, we know that they are strong tissue irritants. Nevertheless, teratology testing of phthalate has been carried out by intraperitoneal injection in doses of 10 g/kg Under these conditions, a chemical peritonitis develops. The animal is in acute pain, massive ascites soon follows and the animal is clearly seriously ill. We're told that, under these conditions, we have the ideal situation for the transfer of phthalates through the uterus into the fetus and that the teratogenic effects so produced are an indication of the hazards to man stemming from phthalates. Now this is the kind of amateurish performance and thinking about which I would like to see something done. I'm sure our speakers would agree that, if the mother is made sick by the conditions of the test, one has to be cautious about the interpretation of the result. Yet, we have no clear statement of this fact in any guideline. No official recognition of the need for caution of this sort is made and the great number of amateurs who've latched onto this field as consumer advocates and do-gooders are not cognizant of these elementary facts.

DR. LAYTON: I agree with Dr. Golberg's statement. I spoke only of drugs and I am glad that I'm backed into that corner because at least with a drug, we can weigh the risk of giving the drug against not giving the drug and Dr. Kelsey has already talked about that, saying that drugs for treating leukemia might almost be assumed to be teratogenic. But there are problems that are not scientific when we talk about other environmental agents. As you point out, people in the field who don't know much about it exert inappropriate pressure on agencies like the FDA.

CAROLE A. KIMMEL (Harvard Medical School, Boston, Massachusetts): I'd like to say that the human case report we mentioned (*Teratology 4*, 15, 1971) is the one and only report that I know of where salicylates were determined in the offspring after injecting salicylates during pregnancy. As that was done late in pregnancy, it doesn't really correlate with any teratogenic work that we've done. One point that I would like to make is that when the salicylates are administered to rats, a fairly large dose is required to produce any effect. However, if you look at the plasma levels in the animal, you see that with the large dose, such as 500 mg/kg, the plasma level is the same as that aimed for in patients with rheumatoid arthritis. Further, we have also shown that the teratogenic effects of lower doses of salicylates in rats can be enhanced by other agents such as the administration of therapeutic doses of iron. Dr. Butcher at the Children's Hospital in Cincinnati showed that behavioral or learning defects can be caused in offspring of animals which were treated with extremely low doses of salicylates, such as 125 mg/kg, after enhancement with iron. As plasma levels are a good indicator of the effect on the animal, they should be considered as another parameter in looking at the teratogenic agents. Experimental animals are similar to man in the way that they handle salicylates except that they excrete them four times faster. So, it takes a larger dose to produce similar plasma levels than in man.

DR. LAYTON: I didn't mean to imply that salicylate is not a human teratogen. I don't know. The data certainly suggest that it might be. I would also agree with your idea about blood levels being important. On the other hand, Dr. Wilson (*Fed. Proc. 30,* 104, 1971) has compared data from monkeys with rat data showing that in a rat an equivalent dose teratogenically speaking, was 250 mg/kg as a single dose and 250 mg/kg/day in the monkey for 6 days, so that I think there are some discrepancies. I think the data he got was important, however. It might be possible, in the case of a safe drug like aspirin, to obtain some better data from humans ourselves with the number of therapeutic abortions being done. It wouldn't be too difficult to give a therapeutic dose of aspirin before and see how much they find in the conceptus. I certainly agree that this compound is a possible teratogen.

BERNARD A. BECKER (University of Iowa, Iowa City, Iowa): I would have been much happier to have made my comment before Dr. Golberg made his. I could then have had the opportunity to make a plea for common sense and good science in teratology testing procedures. In response to Dr. Layton's comment, it does not necessarily negate your results because someone turns up a metabolite. Indeed, in the case of diphenylhydantoin, which is metabolized in the mouse primarily to 5'-parahydroxy-phenylhydantoin, the hydroxylated derivative, one gets a zero in terms of teratology or almost zero. This type of biotransformation takes place in rat, dog, man and in the mouse. The possibility of the mouse being more susceptible as a species to demonstrate this effect and not the others, depends, perhaps, on the fact that the mouse metabolized diphenylhydantoin slowly, compared to the other species and the parent compound although ultimately metabolized to a large measure, is present in the maternal animal for a long time. The fact that if one inhibits the metabolism by use of SKF-525A in the pretreatment, one can show an enhancement of the teratogenicity supports this idea. Now may I ask a question of Dr. Kelsey? Can you give me an example of where multigeneration tests turned up some useful information? I can think of two examples in which it was found that the grandaughters of the original treated animals turned out to be of lighter body weight.

DR. KELSEY: We have virtually dropped multigeneration tests as a requirement in drug testing.

JAMES R. BEALL (Schering Corporation, Lafayette, New Jersey): I have two preliminary statements that I would like to make public. Most of the experimental work which has been done on compounds for which details of mechanisms of action are well known and have been on the market for many years. Unfortunately, as we just heard about aspirin, it is difficult to have this amount of data available during the development procedures. I do believe that, since thalidomide, there have been no drugs which have been introduced which have been shown to be teratogenic in humans, at least in the United States. The success of this may, in part, be due to the experimental procedures which many pharmaceutical companies employ. In scanning the PDR, I notice warnings on all compounds to pregnant women. At what point in the development of a drug does the FDA believe that it may not be harmful and give it to women of child bearing age? What sort of data would they like to have to bring that particular warning into proper perspective?

DR. KELSEY: Well, quite frankly, this is a problem that concerns us, too. It's difficult to get enough data to say, with confidence, that a certain adverse effect may only occur once in 10,000 or 50,000 times. This whole question is now under active consideration with us.

SECTION VI

THE INCORPORATION OF TERATOGENIC AGENTS INTO THE MAMMALIAN EMBRYO

Richard G. Skalko
David S. Packard, Jr.*

The persistent and ever-increasing awareness of the hazards of a wide variety of environmental chemicals is well known and concern about these hazards transcends the usual objectivity of scientific investigations. This has made the study of environmental toxicology the subject of scrutiny not only by regulatory agencies and legislative bodies but, through the communications media, it has become an area of awareness by the general public. Certainly the recent history of many environmental chemicals, e.g., thalidomide, sodium cyclamate, methyl mercury, DDT, 2,4,5–T and its contaminant dioxin, and hexachlorophene, has made the scientific community, industry and the lay public aware of the necessity to develop testing procedures which are scientifically valid and which can define limits of risk to the human organism.[33,55]

Among the possible toxic responses of vertebrates is the ability of both therapeutic and environmental chemicals to produce developmental defects in embryos due to exposure during critical periods of gestation. In mammals, this "teratogenic potential" is based upon two interrelated assumptions: first, these compounds cross the placenta and are capable of affecting the cells of the developing embryo *directly*; or second, they may alter the physiology of the pregnant female primarily and produce their developmental effects *indirectly*.[31] A corollary to these assumptions, which has gained impetus in recent years, is that alterations in maternal physiology can impair normal catabolic processes and result in an increase in placental transfer of a teratogen, and a corresponding increase in the observed teratogenic effect. Thus, the natural pyrimidines thymidine, thymine and uracil, when given simultaneously with the halogenated analog 5-fluorouracil, enhance the teratogenic effects of the latter compound.[7,66] The site of interaction between the normal metabolite and teratogen appears to be the maternal liver, as thymine

*Department of Anatomy, State University of New York-Upstate Medical Center, Syracuse, New York.

inhibits catabolism of 5-fluorouracil by the soluble enzyme pyrimidine dehydrogenase. This inhibition results in higher serum levels of the teratogen and prolonged availability time to the embryo.[47] Similarly, SKF-525A (β-diethylaminoethyl diphenylpropyl acetate), a compound that inhibits liver microsomal enzymes, enhances the teratogenicity of cyclophosphamide in mice while phenobarbital, an inducer of similar enzyme systems, interferes with the teratogenic response.[12] This variation in biological response is related to the ability of SKF-525A to increase, and phenobarbital to reduce, both the availability time and levels of cyclophosphamide which reach the embryo.[13] The studies cited above offer strong presumptive evidence that the ability of most chemical teratogens to produce congenital malformations *in vivo* is the result of two factors: 1) the availability time of the compound and 2) its effective concentration in the embryo.

In recent years, many experimental methods have been employed to both demonstrate the localization of teratogens within the mammalian embryo, and to amplify the concept of stage specificity[63] by defining, within fairly precise limits, how long the compound is available for placental transport. These studies are an essential prelude to the development of an accurate model system to understand the cellular and chemical mechanisms of teratogenic action. As emphasized by Karnofsky,[24]

> "Progress in understanding the teratogenic effects of a drug will come from a systematic exploration of all of the involved factors...in several species. The mechanism of action of a drug on a subcellular, cellular and organ level will be related to detailed information on maternal physiology, placental function and embryological development for each species. If this is done for several important drugs, model systems can be constructed from which the factors involved in producing fetal abnormalities can be interpreted and weighed."

This selective review of the current status of knowledge about maternal metabolism, placental transport and localization in the conceptus of a variety of known and suspected teratogens is presented in order that this information may serve as the first step in the definition of the mechanism of action of these compounds *in situ*. We reaffirm the view that to understand how teratogens act, the paramount responsibility of an investigator is to define specific cellular populations within the embryo that are affected. To make this definition, it is necessary to demonstrate that the compound in question reaches the embryo in measurable amounts during a teratogenic event.

Thalidomide

Thalidomide is one of a very small group of documented human teratogens.[29] This compound is teratogenic in the rhesus monkey,[65] and the rabbit,[45] but poorly so in rats.[3] When either rabbits or rats are administered 10 mg/kg ^{3}H-thalidomide orally in 0.5% carboxymethylcellulose, plasma levels are maximal at 1 hour (rabbit) and 3 hours (rat). After reaching their maxima, the decline is similar in both species, with an estimated $t_{1/2}$ of 3 hours.[46] In the rhesus monkey, administration of 10 mg/kg in dimethylsulfoxide (DMSO) results in a peak plasma concentration at 3 hours, with a decline from this peak being similar to that in the other two species, having a $t_{1/2}$ of 3 hours.[48] When the dosage of ^{3}H-thalidomide is increased to 50 mg/kg, there is a corresponding shift in peak plasma concentrations to 6 hours. In view of the fact that there are species differences in liver metabolism of this teratogen, the differences in peak plasma concentrations may be misleading. However, the demonstration of dose-dependent differences in the rhesus indicates that one of the criteria for enhances teratogenic effect, change in availability time, is certainly operative in this species. That thalidomide enters the embryo or fetus has been demonstrated for both the rabbit[10] and the mouse.[57]

Diphenylhydantoin

An anti-epileptic drug, diphenylhydantoin (dilantin), is teratogenic in mice[15] and rats.[18] It reaches a peak plasma concentration at one hour after administration and is detectable at significant levels in pregnant animals at 24 hours.[62] There is a rapid equilibrium between mother and fetus after one hour and the drug can be localized primarily in the myocardium, liver, intestine and adrenal of both organisms with no preferential localization in neural tissues.[59] Harbison and Becker[16] have shown that SKF-525A enhances the teratogenic effects of diphenylhydantoin with a coincident increase in the availability time of this compound as measured in maternal plasma, placenta and fetus. In the fetus, there is a shift in peak concentration from one hour to eight hours after injection. When phenobarbital is used, the reverse occurs, i.e., reduction of embryotoxicity and decrease in availability time.[17]

Methadone

This compound, now being widely used as a heroin substitute in humans, has been shown to be free of some of the pregnancy-related side effects of heroin addiction, especially the lack of withdrawal symptoms by the neonate.[60] There are no documented teratogenic effects of this drug in rats and rabbits[32] although the compound freely crosses the rat placenta and is randomly distributed throughout the fetus.[35]

237

Tetrahydrocannabinol

This compound, the main psychoactive ingredient of marihuana, has embryotoxic and teratogenic potential in a variety of animal species. In mice, where this compound is mainly embryocidal, peak maternal plasma concentrations are observed one to five hours after administration as they are in both placenta and fetus.[19]

Salicylates

The salicylate compounds, sodium salicylate and acetylsalicylic acid are teratogenic in rats,[61,25] mice[26] and the rhesus monkey.[64] In the rat, Kimmel, Wilson and Schumacher[25] have shown that the concentration of injected aspirin peaks at 3 hours and is detectable up to 24 hours later in both maternal serum and embryo. If the animals are pretreated with benzoic acid, the teratogenic effect of aspirin is potentiated. Under these conditions, no concentration peak is observed but a high concentration is maintained between 3 and 12 hours after administration in both maternal serum and embryo. In mice, there is a definite strain difference with respect to embryolethality but none with respect to rib malformations.[27] In contrast, however, there is no difference between the strains in the distribution of ^{14}C-salicylic acid in maternal liver, blood or fetus up to 4 hours after administration. Salicylate or pentobarbital pre-treatment, both of which are capable of decreasing the frequency of salicylate-induced fetal damage, were also without effect in altering the distribution of the labeled compound.[9]

Glucocorticoids

Since the initial demonstration by Kalter[23] that there are distinct strain differences in the teratogenic response of mice to cortisone, numerous studies have documented the genetic basis for this differential susceptibility.[11] Other glucocorticoids show this phenomenon,[68] and the cellular mechanisms responsible for the ability of these compounds to produce cleft palate are discussed elsewhere in this symposium.[28] Levine, et al.,[30] showed that, in two strains of mice sensitive (A/Jax) and resistant (CBA) to the teratogenic action of cortisone, more of the compound was detected in the fetuses of the sensitive strain, In addition, the rate of disappearance of ^{14}C-cortisol was faster in the resistant strain. Their data suggested that while placental transport was not different, there were more likely differences in metabolism and/or binding by the fetuses of the two strains to account for the differences in cleft palate susceptibility. Support for this interpretation has come from a more rigorous analysis of triamcinolone as the teratogen in three strains with different cleft palate sensitivities, A/Jax, C3H and CBA.[69] The most resistant of the three, (CBA), metabolized the drug faster than the other two, although levels of

238

the unmetabolized drug in maternal livers of all strains were not significantly different. As with cortisone, the level of triamcinolone in the fetus of the CBA strain was 60% of that found in the other two. Of practical importance to future studies along the lines outlined in this communication was the observation that no differences between the intermediate (C3H) and sensitive (A/Jax) strains could be detected as far as distribution in placenta or embryo nor in their ability to metabolize triamcinolone. That triamcinolone itself, and not a metabolite, is the teratogen has been documented,[68] and is consistent with other studies which have shown both thalidomide[46] and trypan blue[1] to be the active agent in susceptible species.

Attempts to define susceptible cell populations in the developing palate with autoradiography have met with equivocal results. While radioactively labeled cortisone has been localized in the palatine shelves of mouse embryos,[56,67] there is neither evidence of a preferential localization nor a difference in distribution between embryos of the same litter. There is also no difference in the distribution of teratogenic and non-teratogenic cortical steroids using this method.[58]

Other Teratogens

Many teratogens have been localized in the embryo and/or fetus of susceptible species. Among those of current interest in the study of teratogenic mechanisms are actinomycin,[22] hydroxyurea,[49] 6-azauridine,[14] ethionine[44] and 5-fluorouracil.[8,47]

The Halogenated Deoxyribonucleosides

The halogenated analogs of deoxyuridine and thymidine are teratogenic when administered to pregnant animals. These include FUdR,[34] ClUdR,[4] BUdR[53] and IUdR.[54,3] The structural relationship between the van der Waal's radii of the halogens to that of either the 5-hydrogen or 5-methyl groups of the normal metabolites (Fig. 1) suggests that the latter three compounds may produce their biological effect by serving as thymidine analogs.[37] An essential corollary to this interpretation is that, to be effective, these compounds must be incorporated into DNA and, with one exception,[43] this appears to be so.[6,40]

Over the past few years, our laboratory has been involved in a systematic analysis of two of the thymidine analogs, BUdR and IUdR, as teratogens in mice. On day 10 (stage 18) of gestation, these compounds produce quantitatively different developmental effects, IUdR being more toxic in terms of embryolethality (Table 1). The teratogenic response is qualitatively similar, however, as 1000 mg/kg BUdR and 300 mg/kg IUdR produce 100% and 95% cleft palate, respectively, in survivors. While not conclusive, this

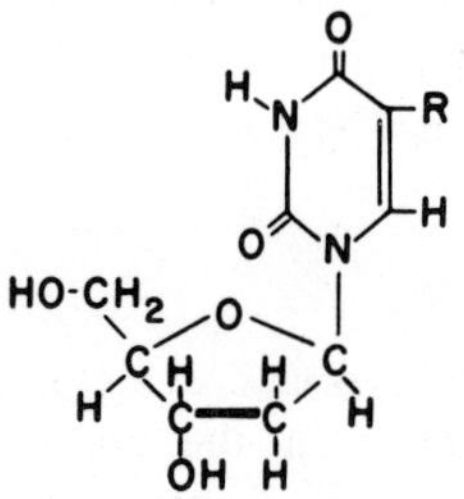

R	van der Waals' Radii (A°)	COMPOUND
(H)	1.2	UdR
(F)	1.35	FUdR
(Cl)	1.80	CUdR
(Br)	1.95	BUdR
(CH₃)	2.0	TdR
(I)	2.15	IUdR

Figure 1. Structural relationship between thymidine, deoxyuridine and their halogenated analogs. (From Prusoff, *et al.,* 1965; reprinted with permission of the author and the New York Academy of Sciences.)

TABLE 1

Teratogenic Response of the Day 10 (Stage 18) Mouse Embryo to BUdR and IUdR

Compound	Dose (mg/kg)	No. of Litters	No. of Sites	Resorptions		Survivors With					
						Polydactyly		Ectrodactyly		Cleft Palate	
				No.	%	No.	%	No.	%	No.	%
BUdR	300	10	113	7	6	7	7	—	—	8	8
	500	11	132	9	7	20	16	—	—	38	31
	1000	10	130	3	2	21	16	48	37	127	100
IUdR	300	10	105	48	46	9	16	10	18	54	95
	500	11	137	126	92	—	—	—	—	4	36

similarity of response suggested to us that there may also be similar sites and mechanisms of action between the two compounds. In order to narrow down the presumed site of action, we performed three interrelated experiments. First, we studied *availability time* of both the natural metabolite (TdR) and the analogs; second, the *kinetics of nucleoside incorporation into DNA* in embryo and placenta with all 3 compounds at trace doses and the analogs at teratogenic doses and, finally, the *cellular localization* of the compounds in maternal intestine and embryo.

For all experiments, the 10-day (stage 18) mouse embryo was used. The first two studies were combined in the same protocol so that availability time and incorporation kinetics were analyzed simultaneously in the same litter. For trace experiments, pregnant females were administered 200 μCi/kg of either 6-^{3}H-TdR, 6-^{3}H-BUdR or 6-^{3}H-IUdR (all compounds supplied by Schwarz-Mann, Orangeburg, New York) and killed at intervals between 15 min. and 4 hr. after injection. Embryos and placentas were removed separately, placed in cold 0.5M PCA (perchloric acid), weighed and homogenized. The acid-soluble fractions were collected and DNA extracted from the precipitate.[42] To determine if the radioactivity in the acid-soluble fraction represented nucleotide and not catabolic byproducts of pyrimidine metabolism, advantage was taken of the fact that nucleotides adsorb quantitatively to activated charcoal.[20] By calculating the difference between the amount of activity in an aliquot of the acid-soluble fraction and the amount not adsorbed to activated charcoal, we arrived at a value of estimated nucleotide (precursor) activity (Table 2). There are some differences between the three compounds when they are administered in trace doses, however, definite similarities exist. Peak levels of all compounds in the placenta occur at the first time point studied, and drop to low or unmeasurable values between 1 and 4 hours after injection. In the embryo, peak activity occurred at 15-30 min. (TdR, BUdR) or at 30 min. (IUdR). Peak specific activity in the DNA fraction occurred at one hour after injection in both placenta and embryo (Fig. 2, Fig. 3). That our method for analyzing the availability of the precursor is valid, is suggested by many studies which indicate that TdR availability *in vivo* is on the order of 30 min. to 2 hr.[36,5] On the other hand, . if ^{32}P is used as the isotopic precursor for DNA synthesis, measurable amounts are detected in the acid-soluble fractions of placenta and embryo up to 8 hours after injection and peak incorporation into DNA occurs at 6 hrs.[52]

When teratogenic doses of BUdR (500 mg+200 μCi/kg) or IUdR (300 mg+200 μCi/kg) are used, no change is observed in the kinetics of ^{3}H-BUdR nucleotide in the placenta, although a demonstrable peak occurs at 30 min. with ^{3}H-IUdR (Table 3). These dosages result in a shift in peak nucleotide specific activity in the embryo to 30 min. (BUdR) and 30—60 min.

TABLE 2

Specific Activity of the Nucleotide Fraction of Placenta and Embryo After
Administration of Trace Doses of Labeled Nucleoside

PLACENTA

Time (hr.)	6-^{3}H-TdR*	6-^{3}H-BUdR	6-^{3}H-IUdR
0.25	119.2 ± 10.1 [†]	104.9 ± 13.6	93.6 ± 14.3
0.50	68.8 ± 5.5	63.9 ± 9.8	89.8 ± 6.9
1.00	25.2 ± 3.9	44.7 ± 15.6	43.1 ± 10.0
2.00	26.1 ± 11.9		20.0 ± 9.5
4.00	22.3 ± 7.9		

EMBRYO

Time (hr.)	6-^{3}H-TdR*	6-^{3}H-BUdR	6-^{3}H-IUdR
0.25	79.9 ± 18.3	51.4 ± 19.8	41.2 ± 7.5
0.50	71.3 ± 13.2	38.1 ± 14.1	75.3 ± 7.8
1.00	57.4 ± 27.3	49.9 ± 10.8	39.9 ± 7.7
2.00	34.5 ± 11.2		54.6 ± 25.1
4.00	36.9 ± 11.0		5.8 ± 2.5

* all compounds administered at a dose of 200 μCi/kg.

[†] mean dpm(x10^3)/g wet weight ± S.E.

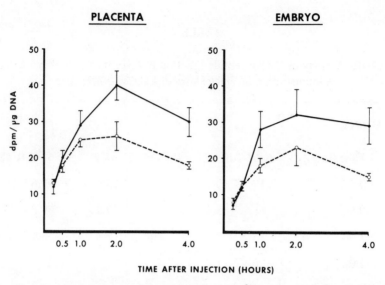

Figure 2. Incorporation of trace doses of 6-^{3}H-TdR and 6-^{3}H-BUdR into the DNA of placenta and embryo. (●——● = TdR; ○-----○ = BUdR)

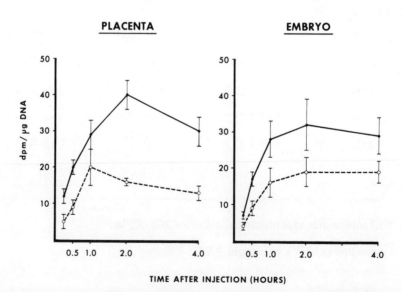

Figure 3. Incorporation of trace doses of 6-^{3}H-TdR and 6-^{3}H-IUdR into the DNA of placenta and embryo. (●——● = TdR; ○-----○ = IUdR)

TABLE 3

Specific Activity of the Nucleotide Fraction of Placenta and Embryo After Administration of Teratogenic Doses of 6-^{3}H-BUdR or 6-^{3}H-IUdR.

PLACENTA

Time (hr.)	6-^{3}H-BUdR*	6-^{3}H-IUdR
0.25	122.6 $\pm$ 31.5 †	146.6 $\pm$ 8.9
0.50	104.3 $\pm$ 8.1	236.6 $\pm$ 54.0
1.00	48.7 $\pm$ 10.6	113.1 $\pm$ 14.4
2.00	37.4 $\pm$ 17.3	47.2 $\pm$ 6.2
4.00	33.4 $\pm$ 25.9	31.2 $\pm$ 1.0

EMBRYO

0.25	76.5 $\pm$ 1.8	80.7 $\pm$ 1.0
0.50	101.8 $\pm$ 12.7	105.7 $\pm$ 7.8
1.00	77.3 $\pm$ 15.0	117.3 $\pm$ 22.9
2.00	69.3 $\pm$ 20.2	59.8 $\pm$ 15.1
4.00	8.5 $\pm$ 2.8	41.0 $\pm$ 6.8

*6-^{3}H-BUdR administered as 200 μCi + 500 mg/kg; 6-^{3}H-IUdR administered as 200 μCi + 300 mg/kg.

†mean dpm (x10^3)/g wet weight $\pm$ S.E.

(IUdR), although activity then declines to levels at the limits of resolution of the method by 4 hr. No change was observed with respect to incorporation of these compounds into the DNA of the placenta. In the embryo, however, the change in nucleotide kinetics is reflected in a shift in incorporation maxima from 1 to 2 hr. for both compounds (Fig. 4).

To determine if the radioactivity present in the DNA fraction represented unchanged halogenated base (BU or IU), the DNA fractions from selected experiments were hydrolyzed to their constituent bases.[21] The bases were then analyzed by thin-layer chromatography on MN-300 cellulose sheets, using thymine, bromouracil and iodouracil as standards, in a solvent system consisting of methanol: HCl: H_2O (65: 17: 18 v/v). The resultant Rf's (Table 4) are in close agreement with those described by Randerath and Randerath[39] using the same solvent but in different proportions. Neither BU nor IU were detectable as UV-absorbing spots with this method. If, however, carrier amounts of BU or IU were added to the DNA hydrolysates, and the areas corresponding to these compounds eluted with 0.1N HCl, it was found that the bulk (> 80%) of the radioactivity present co-chromatographed with the carrier compound.

To determine cellular localization of TdR, BUdR and IUdR in the embryo, randomly selected pregnant females were administered 200 μCi/kg of the specific labeled compound. Two hours after injection, the animals were killed and segments of maternal intestine together with the embryos were removed, fixed in cold ethanol: acetic acid (3:1), and processed for auto-radiography. Irrespective of the pyrimidine nucleoside used, the cellular localization was identical. In the intestine labeled cells were restricted to the crypts of Lieberkühn.[38] In the embryo, cell labeling was extensive but, in the neural epithelium, label was restricted to the lateral region of the primitive ependymal zone.[51] Representative micrographs are shown in Plate 1.

Collectively, these studies indicate that BUdR and IUdR act as thymidine analogs at a time when they are exerting a teratogenic influence on the mouse embryo. In spite of the documented observations from many laboratories that the developmental effects of BUdR *in vitro* are related to its role as a thymidine analog and that incorporation into DNA is an essential pre-requisite,[2,6] it is difficult to state with absolute certainty that incorporation into DNA is equivalent to teratogenesis. For one thing, all cells capable of DNA synthesis incorporate BUdR and IUdR during the availability time. It is obvious from our teratogenic data, however, that not all cells are equally affected. It may well be that, at any specific time in development, the embryo is a mosaic of the two cell types, those sensitive and those tolerant to the influence of the halogenated nucleosides.[53] For these teratogens, and many others mentioned in this review, the next logical step in determining the

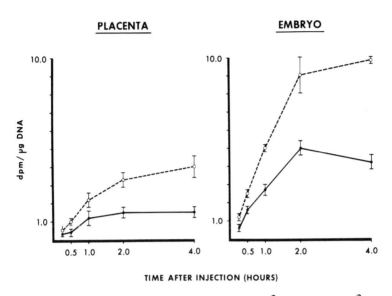

Figure 4. Incorporation of teratogenic doses of 6-³H-BUdR and 6-³H-IUdR into the DNA of placenta and embryo. Specific details described in the text. (●——● = BUdR; ○-----○ = IUdR)

TABLE 4

R_f Values of the Pyrimidine Bases Used in this Study. Analytical Details Described in the Text.

COMPOUND	R_f
Thymine	0.79
Bromouracil	0.73
Iodouracil	0.72

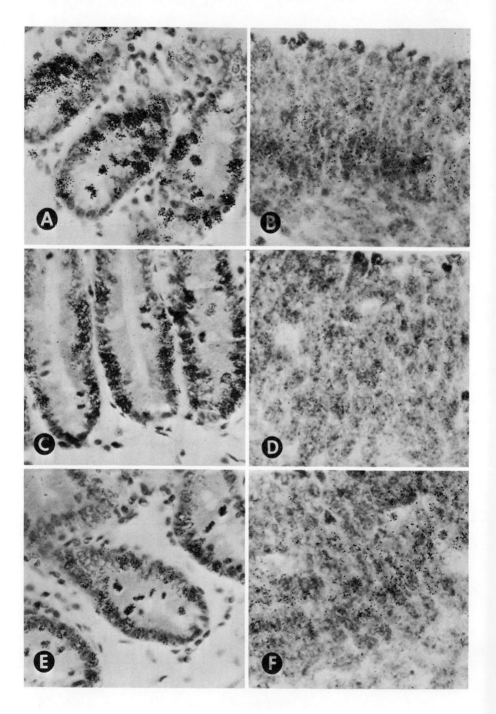

PLATE 1

All photomicrographs were taken with a Zeiss Photomicroscope II, 590nm interference filter, 500x. Details are described in the text.

A – 6-^{3}H-TdR.   maternal intestine

B – 6-^{3}H-TdR.   embryo neural tube

C – 6-^{3}H-BUdR.   maternal intestine

D – 6-^{3}H-BUdR.   embryo neural tube

E – 6-^{3}H-IUdR.   maternal intestine

F – 6-^{3}H-IUdR.   embryo neural tube

quantitative aspects of teratogenesis may be to define the sensitive cell types. Having determined that many teratogens cross the placenta and can be localized within the embryo is, in our view, a necessary prelude to localization of sensitive cells. Perhaps the entire key to unraveling how teratogens act is to determine not only quantitative alterations in a number of biochemical parameters, but to assay the formation of cell-specific products (e.g., collagen, myosin, acid mucoproteins), study alterations of cell-to-cell relationships and relate these to changes in cell morphology. Of particular interest in this regard is the recent report of Seegmiller, Overman and Runner[50] where 6-aminonicotinamide-induced micromelia in chick embryos results from specific degenerative changes in central chondrogenic cells in the developing limb.

Summary and Conclusions

The ground work for the studies outlined in this review was provided many years ago by Runner and Dagg[41] when they asked four interrelated questions relative to the responsiveness of the embryo to teratogens. These were:

> "1. At what stage is the influence effective?
> 2. What is the duration of action of the influence?
> 3. Where within the embryo is the responsive site?
> 4. How much recovery or repair is possible?"

In the ensuing twelve years, it has not been possible to answer all of these questions for all teratogens. However, by determining the kinetics of placental transport, we are close to having answers to the first two and by directing attention to sensitive cell populations, we will be able to eventually answer the latter two. Once this has been accomplished for many teratogens, it will then be possible to study the cellular, chemical and organismal basis for dose-response phenomena. It is only with a rational and quantitative explanation of what dose-response means in developing systems that we may one day arrive at an understanding of potential human risk for a variety of chemical compounds.

ACKNOWLEDGEMENTS

The authors express their appreciation to Allen M. Niles, Carol A. Cooper, Robert D. Sax, Donna A. Caniano and Don Driscoll for their assistance in various aspects of this work.

REFERENCES

1. A.R. Beaudoin and M.J. Pickering, *Anat. Rec. 137,* 297, 1960.

2. R. Bischoff and H. Holtzer, *J. Cell Biol. 44,* 134, 1970.

3. R. Cahen, *Clin. Pharmacol. Ther. 5,* 480, 1964.

4. S. Chaube and M.L. Murphy, *Cancer Res. 24,* 1896, 1964.

5. J.E. Cleaver, Thymidine Metabolism and Cell Kinetics, American Elsevier, New York, 1967.

6. A.W. Coleman, J.R. Coleman, D. Kankel and I. Werner, *Exp. Cell Res. 59,* 319, 1970.

7. C.P. Dagg and E. Kallio, *Anat. Rec. 142,* 301, 1962.

8. C.P. Dagg, A. Doerr and C. Offutt, *Biol. Neonat. 10,* 32, 1966.

9. M. Eriksson and K.S. Larsson, *Acta Pharmacol. et Toxicol. 29,* 256, 1971.

10. S. Fabro, H. Schumacher, R.L. Smith and R.T. Williams, *Nature 201,* 1125, 1964.

11. F.C. Fraser, this Symposium, p. 17.

12. J.E. Gibson and B.A. Becker, *Teratology 1,* 393, 1968.

13. J.E. Gibson and B.A. Becker, *J. Pharmacol. Exp. Therap. 177,* 256, 1971.

14. M.J. Elis and H. Raskova, *Neoplasma 18,* 529, 1971.

15. R.D. Harbison and B.A. Becker, *Teratology 2,* 305, 1969.

16. R.D. Harbison and B.A. Becker, *J. Pharmacol. Exp. Therap. 175,* 283, 1970.

17. R.D. Harbison and B.A. Becker, *Toxicol. Appl. Pharmacol. 20,* 573, 1971.

18. R.D. Harbison and B.A. Becker, *Toxicol. Appl. Pharmacol. 22,* 193, 1972.

19. R.D. Harbison and B. Mantilla-Plata, *J. Pharmacol. Exp. Therap. 180,* 446, 1972.

20. R.B. Hurlbert, *in* Methods in Enzymology, vol. III, S. Colowick and N. Kaplan (Eds.), Academic Press, New York, p. 785, 1957.

251

21. A. Hershey, J. Dixon and M. Chase, *J. Gen. Physiol. 36,* 777, 1953.

22. R.L. Jordan and J.G. Wilson, *Anat. Rec.168,* 549, 1970.

23. H. Kalter, *Genetics 39,* 185, 1954.

24. D. Karnofsky, *Ann. Rev. Pharmacol. 5,* 447, 1965.

25. C.A. Kimmel, J.G. Wilson and H. Schumacher, *Teratology 4,* 15, 1971.

26. K.S. Larsson, H. Bostrom and B. Ericson, *Acta Paediat. Scand. 52,* 36, 1963.

27. K.S. Larsson and M. Eriksson, *Acta Paediat. Scand. 55,* 569, 1966.

28. K.S. Larsson, this Symposium, p. 255.

29. W. Lenz, *Lancet 1,* 45, 1962.

30. A. Levine, S.J. Yaffe and N. Back, *Proc. Soc. Exp. Biol. Med. 129,* 86, 1968.

31. J.B. Lloyd and F. Beck, *in* Lysosomes in Biology and Pathology, J.T. Dingle and H.B. Fell (Eds.), John Wiley, New York, v.1, ch. 16, 1969.

32. J.K. Markham, J.L. Emerson and N.V. Owen, *Nature 233,* 342, 1971.

33. N. Nelson, J.M. Coon, L. Friedman, R. Gosselin, C.M. Kumin, T.A. Loomis, P. Shubik, J.L. Whittenberger and J.G. Wilson, *Toxicol. Appl. Pharmacol. 16,* 264, 1970.

34. K. Ohmuri, *Teratology 5,* 71, 1972.

35. M.A. Peters, M. Turnbow and D. Buchenauer, *J. Pharmacol. Exp. Therap. 181,* 273, 1972.

36. V.R. Potter, *in* The Kinetics of Cellular Proliferation, F. Stollman (Ed.), Grune and Stratton, New York, p. 104, 1959.

37. W.H. Prusoff, Y.S. Bakhle and L. Sekely, *Ann. N.Y. Acad. Sci. 130,* 135, 1965.

38. H. Quastler and F.G. Sherman, *Exp. Cell Res. 17,* 420, 1959.

39. K. Randerath and E. Randerath, *in* Methods in Enzymology, vol. XII, L. Grossman and K. Moldave (Eds.), Academic Press, New York,

p. 323, 1968.

40. R.M. Rizki and T.M. Rizki, *Experientia 28*, 329, 1972.

41. M.N. Runner and C.P. Dagg, Nat. Cancer Inst. Monograph 2, p. 41, 1960.

42. W. Schneider, *J. Biol. Chem. 161*, 293, 1945.

43. D. Shubert and F. Jacob, *Proc. Nat. Acad. Sci. 67*, 247, 1970.

44. P.W. Schultz, J. Graves and R.L. Schultz, *Arch. Biochem. Biophys. 104*, 387, 1964.

45. H. Schumacher, D.A. Blake, J.M. Gurian and J.R. Gillette, *J. Pharmacol. Exp. Therap. 160*, 189, 1968a.

46. H. Schumacher, D.A. Blake and J.R. Gillette, *J. Pharmacol. exp. Therap. 160*, 201, 1968b.

47. H.J. Schumacher, J.G. Wilson and R.L. Jordan, *Teratology 2*, 99, 1969.

48. H.J. Schumacher, J.G. Wilson, J.F. Terapane and S.L. Rosedale, *J. Pharmacol. Exp. Therap. 173*, 265, 1970.

49. W.J. Scott, E.J. Ritter and J.G. Wilson, *Dev. Biol. 26*, 306, 1971.

50. R.E. Seegmiller, D.O. Overman and M.N. Runner, *Dev. Biol. 28*, 555, 1972.

51. R.L. Sidman, I.L. Miale and N. Feder, *Exp. Neurol. 1*, 322, 1959.

52. R.G. Skalko, *J. Exp. Zool. 160*, 171, 1965.

53. R.G. Skalko, D.S. Packard, Jr., R.N. Schwendimann and J.F. Raggio, *Teratology 4*, 87, 1971.

54. R.G. Skalko and D.S. Packard, Jr., *Experientia 29*, 198, 1973.

55. H. Tuchman-Duplessis, *Teratology 5*, 271, 1972.

56. W.J. Waddell, *Teratology 4*, 355, 1971.

57. W.J. Waddell, *Fed. Proc. 31*, 52, 1972a.

58. W.J. Waddell, *Teratology 5*, 219, 1972b.

59. W.J. Waddell and B.L. Mirkin, *Biochem. Pharmacol. 21*, 547, 1972.

60. B.E. Wallach, E. Jerez and G. Blinick, *Am. J. Obstet. Gynecol. 105,* 1226, 1969.

61. J. Warkany and E. Takacs, *Am. J. Path. 35,* 315, 1959.

62. B. Westmoreland and N.H. Bass, *Arch. Neurol. 24,* 158, 1971.

63. J.G. Wilson, *in* First International Conference on Congenital Malformations, Lippincott, Philadelphia, p. 187,1961.

64. J.G. Wilson, *Fed. Proc. 30,* 104, 1971.

65. J.G. Wilson and J.A. Gavan, *Anat. Rec. 158,* 99, 1967.

66. J.G. Wilson, R.L. Jordan and H. Schumacher, *Teratology 2,* 91, 1969.

67. N.K. Wood, A.D. Marks, D.P. Schmitz, D.C. Bowman and P.D. Toto, *J. Dental Res. 51,* 67, 1972.

68. E.F. Zimmerman and D. Bowen, *Teratology 5,* 57, 1972a.

69. E.F. Zimmerman and D. Bowen, *Teratology 5,* 335, 1972b.

MECHANISMS OF CLEFT PALATE FORMATION*

K. Sune Larsson

Cleft palate is one of the most common malformations in humans and is often associated with other types of malformations. In some instances we can trace the etiologic factors to chromosomal abnormalities but in most cases cleft palate is multifactorially determined; that is, a number of genetic and environmental factors are involved.[6] In experimental animals the same complicated interaction between genes and environment determines the cleft palate formation. This apparently gives the option of several mechanisms involved in cleft palate formation and rarely can a specific mode of interaction with the normal development be definitely distinguished. In my opinion, animal studies are justified as a means of explaining the pathogenesis of cleft palate in the human since the difficulties of studying the mechanism in human embryos are obvious. Moreover, cleft palate has been the predominant malformation induced in animal studies using some common drugs such as cortisone, chlorocyclizine and diphenylhydantoin or the herbicide 2,4,5-T, and can be expected to be found in many forthcoming tests for teratogenicity of new compounds.[4,8, 9,17,32]

The normal development of the five anatomical entities listed in Fig. 1 have been shown to be impaired in some way in cleft palate formation: 1) the palatine shelves, 2) the tongue, 3) the mandible, 4) the cranial base and 5) the width of the head. In this symposium, I will restrict myself to the discussion of a few possible mechanisms involved in the formation of isolated cleft palate and analyze the role of some of these factors in view of new and contradictory results.

Palatine Shelves

The palatine shelves are developed from the superior lateral wall of the common oral and nasal cavity and grow vertically on either side of the tongue. The

*Supported by grants from S.M.R.C. Stockholm, nr. 14-x and P-993-08.

CLEFT PALATE

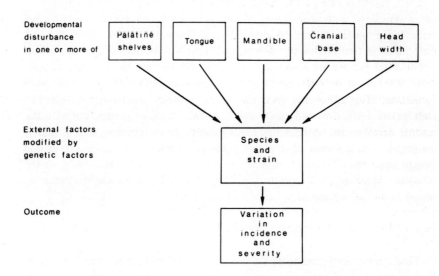

Fig. 1. Principal pathways for cleft palate formation.

256

secondary palate is formed by fusion of the two palatine shelves in a horizontal position above the tongue. The change in position of the shelves from vertical to horizontal is an extremely rapid process; in the mouse embryo it has been shown to take only a few hours.[49] Thus, either failure of the palatine shelves to move from vertical to horizontal position or their failure to fuse could be the cause of cleft palate formation.

What is the evidence for disturbances at palatal closure? With regard to the *epithelium* covering the shelves, there are no indications that a rapid mitotic division in the lateral parts should especially contribute to the change in position of the shelf. A more interesting area is the medial edge of the horizontal shelves. Recent *in vivo* and *in vitro* studies in the mouse indicate that there is a correlation between normal palate formation and spontaneous epithelial cell death in this region and that a cellular contact between palatine shelves is not a prerequisite for midline epithelial disruption.[42] It, therefore, seems quite possible that the mechanism involved in cleft palate is, in some instances, a failure of the epithelium to break down. However, very little is known about which factors can cause this epithelial disturbance *in vivo*. This particular epithelium and its covering substances will probably be of particular interest to many experimental biologists in the near future and be investigated under various conditions.

Most experimental studies indicate an earlier impairment than at the proper fusion and the *mesenchymal* part of the shelves is believed to play its main role in the change of palatal position. Only after the publication of Walker and Fraser's study in 1956[49] could the intermediate stages of transposition of the palatine shelves from the vertical to the horizontal plane be convincingly demonstrated in the mouse embryo. These authors described the rise as a wavelike movement, consisting of a bulging of the medial wall of each palatine shelf, with concurrent regression of the ventral wall. This movement started posteriorly and proceeded in the anterior direction, carrying the shelves into the horizontal position at the same time that the tongue was being forced downwards. It had been assumed that the tongue must first be carried out of the way of the shelves so that the palatine shelves could rapidly rotate upwards as in an erection. Other theories which attempted to explain the change in position of the palatine shelves were a new formation of the shelves directly in the horizontal plane, and a transformation of the shelves by growth in the medial direction over the tongue. Experimental removal of the tongue has shown that in the mouse, in contrast to the rabbit, there is an intrinsic force moving the tongue up into a horizontal position.[51,39]

257

What would be the morphological base in the mesenchymal part of the shelves for the described transposition? The *mesenchymal cells* do not grow rapidly enough to give a plausible explanation nor is there a fiber synthesis which would seem likely to cause such a rapid change of the palatine shelves. On the contrary, substances which inhibit collagen cross-linking and cause a weakening in the connective tissue, produce a high incidence of cleft palate in the rat.[38,43] Mesenchymal cells produce an amorph *ground substance* in addition to fibers. Patten[35] has pointed out that, "...it seems strange that more attention has not been paid to the substratum on which mesenchymal cells must move in the embryonic body." Mucopolysaccharides were, however, identified in the connective tissue of the developing shelves in our early studies on ^{35}S-sulfate incorporation in mouse embryos.[21,22,23,25] It is interesting to compare the autoradiograms showing a high incorporation of ^{35}S-sulfate in the same areas suggested by Patten[35] to be the sites of the most marked movements of the mesenchymal cells (Fig. 2). Based on these studies, I proposed[24] the following theory: "In closure of the secondary palate, (1) the plasticity of the ground substance permits a change in the shape of the fibroblast zones. It can be presumed that (2) changes in the polymerization and/or aggregation of the high-molecular acid mucopolysaccharides and binding of water to them gives rise to tension or changes in pressure in the tissue, resulting in development of a force which causes changes in shape. Consequently, the presence of sulfate-esterified mucopolysaccharides (CSA), with powerful synthesis, in the ground substance of the fibroblast zones is considered to be responsible for the internal force." The expression "internal force" has been created by Walker and Fraser[49] for their description of palatine movement and Lazzaro[27] had already expressed the view that an increase in intercellular substance is responsible for development of a swelling force in the palatine shelves. The presence of sulfated mucopolysaccharides (SMP) in rodents has been confirmed.[2,13,18,19,33,47] An increased synthesis of hyaluronic acid has been demonstrated in the rat palate[37] and histochemical evidence.has been presented for its accumulation in the human palate.[1] Using autoradiography it was possible to demonstrate a decreased sulfation or a diminished production of sulfomucopolysaccharides had taken place during a specified short period of the palatal closure process. Such a change could not be demonstrated with the less sensitive histochemical methods. The change in the sulfomucopolysaccharides of the ground substance was interpreted to result in insufficient development of the internal force in the palatine shelves. Furthermore, it could be assumed that the ability of the palatine shelves to approach each other was decreased after having attained the horizontal plance since the substratum for cell migration in fusion process was changed.

Quantitative measurements of the degree of inhibition of sulfomucopoly-

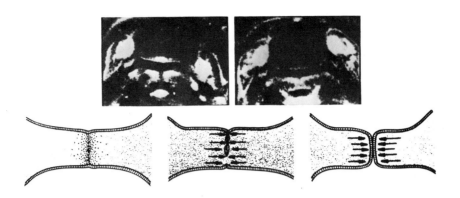

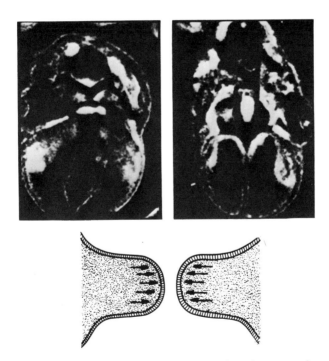

Fig. 2. Comparison between areas suggested to be sites of most marked movements of mesenchymal cells (redrawn from Patten, ref. 35) and auto-radiograms showing high incorporation of ^{35}S-sulfate in palatine shelves of 14- and 15-day-old mouse embryos (ref. 22 and 23).

saccharide synthesis have been made in an attempt to correlate the frequency of clefts induced with cortisol or triamcinolone to their capacity to inhibit SMP synthesis. Zimmerman has claimed, in a series of papers, that there is no such correlation. There are reasons, however, to examine the evidence upon which his conclusion is based.

Figure 3 illustrates the discrepancy in design between my earlier[23] and Andrew and Zimmerman's recent[2] studies on ^{35}S-sulfate incorporation. The preparation period before the shelves change position corresponds to a period of increased SMP synthesis. In my experiments the teratogen cortisone was given on four consecutive days in contrast to a single injection of the teratogens, cortisol or triamcinolone, given in the beginning of the period by Andrew and Zimmerman. The effect of the teratogens on the ^{35}S-sulfate incorporation was also studied during different periods. My studies covered the 48 hours between sulfate injection on day 12 to sacrifice on day 14, representing a substantial part of the palatine shelf preparation period compared to the 1 hour on day 14 studied by Andrew and Zimmerman.[2] The results are summarized in Table 1 which shows that by semiquantitative determination the degree of ^{35}S-sulfate inhibition is evident in both CBA and A/Jax strains. Using scintillation counting, Andrew and Zimmerman showed in the C3H strain that triamcinolone could induce 80 percent clefts already at a 26 percent ^{35}S-sulfate inhibition of labeled sulfate incorporation. Furthermore, cortisol produced only 2 percent clefts at a ^{35}S-sulfate inhibition of 32 percent.

Zimmerman claimed as further evidence that a strain difference in ^{35}S-sulfate incorporation in the sensitive A/Jax strain and in the resistant CBA strain had not been shown.[23] Such a strain difference might exist but the isotope and histochemical methods might not be sensitive enough to demonstrate it. On the other hand, we know from *in vivo* studies that strain differences in frequency of cortisone-induced cleft palates are correlated to the time differences for palatal closure.[50] *In vitro* studies with both CBA and A/Jax strains have shown that hydrocortisone retards the growth and fusion of the palatine shelves, but never prevents their final fusion.[20] Another argument against the role of acid mucopolysaccharide impairment in cleft palate formation was Nanda's studies[33] showing a decreased ^{35}S-sulfate incorporation in the rat palate after cortisone treatment even if it was accepted that this drug could not produce cleft palate in this species. It is a pity that he studied the incorporation over the wrong period, i.e., when the palate was already closed and when the bone formation was in an advanced stage. Recent experiments by Walker[48] have shown, furthermore, that by using various anti-inflammatory drugs it is even possible to produce cleft palate in rats with triamcinolone, betamethasone and dexamethasone, but not with methylprednisolone or cortisone. A combination treatment of cortisone and vitamin A has been per-

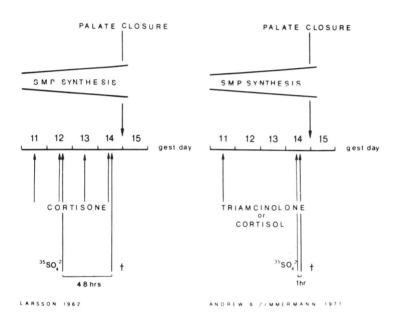

LARSSON 1962
ANDREW & ZIMMERMANN 1971

Fig. 3. Comparison of experimental design in studies on the inhibition of ^{35}S-sulfate incorporation in sulfomucopolysaccharides by glucocorticosteroids (ref. 2 and 23).

TABLE 1

Comparison of experimental results in studies of the inhibition of ^{35}S-sulfate incorporation in sulfomucopolysaccharides by glucocorticosteroids

APPOSITION AUTORADIOGRAPHY
Cortisone

	percent cleft palate	$^{35}SO_4^{-2}$ inhibition
125 mg/kg		
4 A/Jax	100	evident
CBA	20	evident

Larsson 1961

SCINTILLATION COUNTING
Cortisol

	percent cleft palate	$^{35}SO_4^{-2}$ inhibition
C3H		
400 mg/kg	75	–
320	70	65
64	2	32
Triamcinolone		
125 mg/kg	100	–
10	80	26
2	0	–

Andrew & Zimmerman 1971

formed. Since excess vitamin A increases the ^{35}S-sulfate incorporation for 48 hours,[18,19] it was apparently believed by Nanda that the decreased incorporation by cortisone should be counteracted and that vitamin A should be an antidote in cortisone-induced cleft palate. In fact, the cortisone-induced ^{35}S-sulfate inhibition was counteracted by vitamin A, but the teratogenic effect was increased.[33,52] Kochar and Johnson[18] clearly demonstrated that the increased uptake of ^{35}S-sulfate by vitamin A treatment could be due to the formation of heteroptic cartilage in the shelves. The mechanism for cleft palate formation by excess vitamin A treatment could also be a direct change in the plasticity of the palatine shelves preventing their change in position. Much more has to be understood about the two substances' basic interference with mucopolysaccharide synthesis and turnover before we can interpret their mode of teratogenic action in combined treatment. Considering their experimental design, I think that Andrew and Zimmerman[2] drew their conclusions a little too far from their scattered observations when they chose the title, "Glucocorticoid induction of cleft palate in mice; no correlation with inhibition of mucopolysaccharide synthesis."

The Tongue and the Mandible

It is interesting to note how the pendulum in research interests swings back and forth. One good example is the increased interest in the role of the tongue in cleft palate formation. For a long time, it was assumed that the tongue must first be carried out of the way before the shelves could attain the horizontal position: see reviews by Peter,[36] Lazzaro[27] and Humphrey.[12] This displacement of the tongue was believed to occur either as a result of muscular contraction or growth of the tongue or oral cavity. It was assumed that once the tongue had been brought down, the palatine shelves could rapidly rotate upwards as a barn door. However, very vew cases showing this process in the intermediate stages were available.[12] Walker, who along with Fraser[49] had demonstrated that the shelves in the mouse could indeed move over the tongue without its first being lowered, found some evidence ten years later for a possible active role of the tongue at palatal closure.[39] The tongue can theoretically be moved either actively due to reflex contraction of the tongue or to passive withdrawal due to head extension. Some studies have been performed which support the theory that the descent of the tongue is induced by fetal muscular movements and is essential for normal palate closure.[3,12,54] Jacobs[14] tested a variety of muscle relaxants and central nervous system depressants in mice, but no clefts were found.

The descent of the tongue and the growth of the mandible are two closely related factors, however, the role of the lower jaw has scarcely been studied and the results are contradictory. Sicker[41] had stated that there was a sudden growth spurt of the lower jaw in the human prior to descent of the tongue and fusion of the palatine shelves. In rats it was found that the mandible grows in length at an increasingly rapid rate before and during palatal closure and that the increase continues after closure.[53] On the contrary, Humphrey[12] did not find the mandibular growth spurt in human embryos nor did Hart et al.[11] in mice before or during palatal closure. Significantly shortened mandibles in A/Jax fetuses with induced cleft palate have been described by Schwartz and Chaudry.[40]

The Cranial Base

Harris[10] reported that the cranial base is flexed at the onset of palate closure in the mouse and the rat, and that the cranial base is straight when the shelves are fused. This observation of a gradual decrease in angulation of the cranial base during the morphogenesis of the palate has been confirmed by Verrusio[46] and by Hart et al.[11] Moreover, Harris pointed out that the process of palatal closure involved a change in spatial relations between the palatal shelves and the tongue and that the flexed cranial base might give the embryo an additional range of movement in the anterior part of the head. The mechanism for cortisone-induced cleft palate was suggested to be a constriction of the embryo due to reduced amount of amniotic fluid.[10] This hypothesis could not be supported by Fraser et al.[7] since a dose of cortisone that caused cleft palate in about half the embryos, caused the same decrease in amniotic fluid in embryos with and without clefts.

We have also approached the problem of the role of cranial base development in recent studies. In order to investigate the role of the cranial base for normal palate closure we studied autoradiographically the growth by ^{3}H-thymidine and ^{35}S-sulfate incorporation in mice.[29] It was found that the cranial base cartilage has a special kink immediately anterior to the hypophysis before the palatal closure and that the cranial base is straightened out when the shelves are closed normally (Fig. 4). This particular area had the highest mitotic index but the high rate of cell division continued after the palatal closure. This percentage of labeled cells in the expanding area was reduced markedly in fetuses from 6-aminonicotinamide-treated mothers.[29] It is interesting to note that in embryos treated with 6-aminonicotinamide causing a high incidence of isolated cleft palate, the cartilage kink was still present at the time the palate should have been closed.

In order to further analyze whether or not the lack of straightening of the cranial base could be a cause of the cleft palate or if the cleft palate caused the persistence of the cartilage kink, we have undertaken the following experiments.[26] The results so far obtained are shown in Fig. 5 as a comparison of palatal status and cranial base shape in 15-day-old mouse embryos. From

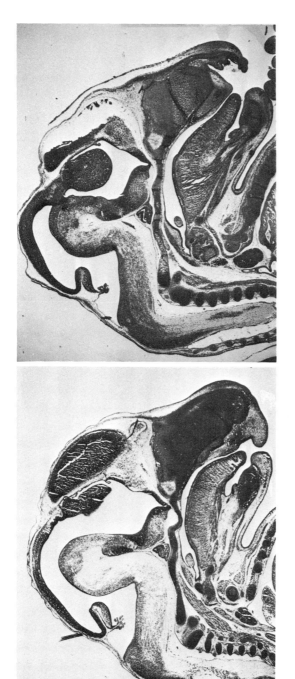

Fig. 4. Sagittal section of 15-day-old mouse embryos. To the left is a cleft palate produced by cortisone treatment; the cranial base shows the particular kink which is characteristic of embryos before palatal closure. To the right is an embryo with a spontaneous cleft lip-palate; the cranial base is straightened out as in embryos with normally closed palate.

265

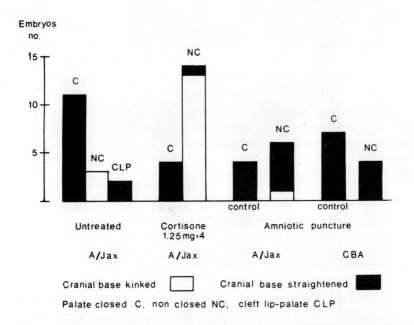

COMPARISON OF PALATE STATUS AND CRANIAL BASE SHAPE

Fig. 5. Comparison of cleft palate status and cranial base shape in normal mouse embryos, after amniotic puncture and in embryos from mothers treated with cortisone for cleft palate formation.

A/Jax untreated mothers, 11 embryos with the palate closed all show a straightened cranial base. The three still nonclosed show the kink. The embryos with cleft lip-palate confirm our earlier observation that in these embryos the cranial base straightens out.[29] After treatment with cortisone in a dose which usually produces cleft palate in 100 percent in the A/Jax strain, however, we got 4 embryos with closed palate. These showed a completely straightened cranial base. Thirteen out of fourteen embryos with nonclosed palate showed the cartilage kink. The one with the straight cranial base and a nonclosed palate could also tentatively be described as an embryo with cleft lip if this latter defect has been small and overlooked. Further analyses of the sections will reveal the type of malformation.

Amniotic puncture was shown in 1956 by Trasler *et al.*[45] to be a good method for production of isolated cleft palate in a high incidence. Due to bending of the head toward the chest, the tongue became a mechanical obstruction for the palatine shelves. As seen from Fig. 5, 11 sham-operated embryos from both A/Jax and CBA strains showed closed palates and straight cranial base. Thus, there was a pure mechanical disturbance by tongue obstruction as a cause for nonclosure of the palate. The cranial base continued to grow and straighten out. The same was true for spontaneous cleft lip-palate embryos (Fig. 4). On the contrary, when a metabolic impairment such as cortisone of 6-aminonicotinamide treatment was used to produce cleft palate there was a retardation of the cranial base development.

Since the changes in cartilage as well as in the palatine shelves occur very rapidly, I find it now even more reasonable to believe in an impairment in the production of intercellular substance in these two entities such as a cleft palate mechanism. It can, therefore, be assumed that many different factors could at any developmental stage prior to the palatal closure cause various cleft palate formation if the damage was severe enough.

Genetic Factors in Cleft Palate Formation

As seen from Figure 1, the influence of external factors can be modified by genetic factors which are expressed in strain and species differences. In attempts to explore various cleft palate mechanisms, the strain and species differences have been of great advantage even though, at the same time, causing some confusion. Some examples from cortisone-induced cleft palate studies in mice will be given.

Kalter[16] showed by reciprocal crosses that the strain differences could be due to maternal influence, in addition to the influence from the embryo's own genetic makeup. In backcrossing experiments he did not find any support for a cytoplasmic factor being responsible for the maternal influence in the susceptible A/Jax strain. Using a nonsurgical method, Marsk *et al.*[31] transferred blastocysts of the A/Jax strain to CBA foster mothers and CBA blastocysts to A/Jax foster mothers. The foster mothers were mated to fertile males of their own strain and recipients were given the 3-day-old blastocysts on day 2. Cortisone, 62.5 mg/kg was given from day 11 for four consecutive days and the embryos were removed on day 16. The difference in eye color made it easy to differentiate the A/Jax and CBA embryos. They were fixed and examined for cleft palate and other abnormalities and their sex was determined. The results are summarized in Fig. 6 and indicate that the matroclinous influence in the A/Jax strain is most likely cytoplasmic. There was no male dominance in the cleft groups, thus excluding a pure x-linked inheritance.[16] Since the autosomal genome must be considered identical in the two crosses, there remain two probable alternatives — cytoplasmic factors inherited through the egg or a uterine influence. The results clearly demonstrated that transferred A/Jax x A/Jax fetuses are not protected in the CBA uterus; they still show 100 percent cortisone-induced cleft palate. The CBA x CBA fetuses in CBA mothers had cleft palate in only 20 percent. Even though we had only a small number of transferred living CBA x CBA fetuses to A/Jax foster mothers, it was clear that there was no real increase in frequency of cleft palate over the original 20 percent for this strain. The A/Jax foster mothers' own fetuses had cleft palate in 100 percent. Thus, the maternal influence observed in the reciprocal crosses cannot be interpreted as uterine.

It is interesting to note that using other strains, SWV and C57B1/10J, for transfer of blastocysts to pseudopregnant foster mothers of the opposite strain and injecting triamcinolone on day 11, Takano et al.[44] found a strong maternal strain influence upon the incidence of cleft palate. In the SWV strain, cleft palates were induced in 39.4 percent and when C57 blastocysts were transferred, 14 out of 40 (35 percent) developed cleft palate. The SWV fetuses had cleft palate in only 11.4 percent (5 out of 44) after transfer, which is very close to the 8.7 percent cleft palate induced in the C57 strain. Unfortunately, no figures for the incidence of the triamcinolone-induced cleft palate were given for reciprocal crosses.

The blastocyst transfer method has, moreover, recently been used[30] in studies on the incorporation of labeled cortisone in CBA and A/Jax embryos. Levine et al.[28] showed that CBA fetuses eliminate ^{14}C-labeled cortisone faster than the A/Jax embryos and suggested that the greater exposure to A/Jax embryos of the teratogen would be the reason for the higher incidence of cortisone-induced cleft palate. Such a strain difference 3 hours after administration of labeled cortisone was also found in our studies. However, when A/Jax x A/Jax embryos were transferred to CBA foster mothers mated to fertile CBA males, the embryos of the two different strains showed the same uptake. Pure strains were used as controls in each separate experiment and the

CORTISONE-INDUCED CLEFT PALATE

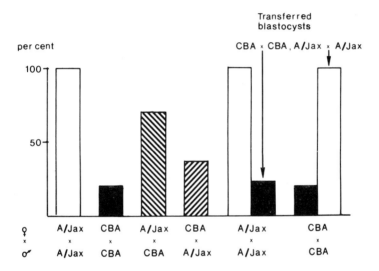

Fig. 6. Strain differences in cortisone-induced cleft palate examined in reciprocal crosses and after blastocyst transfer.

lower uptake in the litters from CBA mothers compared to litters from A/Jax mothers was confirmed. These results and the results of our earlier blastocyst transfer studies indicate that the genetically determined strain difference in susceptibility is not due to a difference in the amount of exposure of the teratogen, which was originally postulated by Levine *et al.* [28] Several isotope studies have been carried out in an attempt to clarify the strain differences in maternal-fetal handling of teratogenic glucocorticosteroids and difference in teratogenic response. [34,35]

Dostal and Jellinek [5] tried intra-amniotic administration of cortisol to avoid differences in maternal handling of the drug and claimed at first that they could not find a difference in cleft palate incidence in different strains. Now they have found such a difference which corroborated our results from experiments with blastocyst transfer. [15]

CONCLUSION

1. Looking for possible mechanisms of cleft palate formation, the particular research interest in disturbances in the developmental palatine shelves compared to other pertinent structures is obvious.

2. Important basic information on the role of the death of the epithelial cells in the midline of the palate for the normal fusion has recently been obtained.

3. Special attention has been paid to the role of the intercellular substance in the mesenchyme of the shelves. Many recent studies seem to further support the hypothesis of an impairment with acid mucopolysaccharide formation in the shelves as a mechanism in cleft palate formation.

4. A similar metabolic disturbance in the developmental cranial base cartilage might be another plausible mechanism for cleft palate formation. This cartilage seems to be of particular interest for further studies on cleft palate mechanisms since it is not changed when cleft palate is induced by mechanical interference with shelf movement in contrast to drug-induced cleft palates.

5. The species and strain differences in susceptibility to various teratogens can be surmised to be of further use in studies on certain modes of cleft palate induction. Embryo transfer between resistant and sensitive strains of mice followed by treatment with a teratogen have been used to study the matroclinous influence on the incidence of cortisone-induced cleft palate. A cytoplasmic factor seems to be responsible for the susceptibility in the A/Jax strain.

ACKNOWLEDGEMENTS

I am greatly indebted to Dr. Barbro Larsson and Mrs. Cheryl Hord for excellent librarian and secretarial assistance.

REFERENCES

1. H. Anderson and M. Mathiessen, *Acta Anat. 68*, 473, 1967.

2. F.D. Andrew and E.F. Zimmerman, *Teratology 4*, 31, 1971.

3. C.S. Borden, *Amer. J. Orthodont. 56*, 531, 1969.

4. K.D. Courtney, D.W. Gaylor, M.D. Hogan, H.L. Falk, R.R. Bates and J. Mitchell, *Science 168*, 864, 1970.

5. M. Dostal and R. Jelinek, *Teratology 4*, 486, 1971.

6. F.C. Fraser, *Fed. Proc. 30*, 100, 1971.

7. F.C. Fraser, D. Chew and A.C. Verrusio, *Nature 214*, 417, 1967.

8. F.C. Fraser and T.D. Fainstat, *Pediatrics 8*, 527, 1951.

9. J.E. Gibson and B.A. Becker, *Proc. Soc. Exp. Biol. Med. 128*, 905, 1968.

10. J.W.S. Harris, *Nature 203*, 533, 1964.

11. J.C. Hart, G.R. Smiley and A.D. Dixon, *Teratology 6*, 43, 1972.

12. T. Humphrey, *Am. J. Anat. 125*, 317, 1969.

13. R.M. Jacobs, *Anat. Rec. 150*, 271, 1964.

14. R.M. Jacobs, *Teratology 4*, 25, 1971.

15. R. Jelinek, Personal communication.

16. H. Kalter, *Genetics 39*, 185, 1954.

17. C.T.G. King, S.A. Weaver and S.A. Narrod, *J. Pharmacol. Exp. Ther. 147*, 391, 1965.

18. D.M. Kochhar and E.M. Johnson, *J. Embryol. Exp. Morph. 14*, 233, 1965.

19. D.M. Kochhar, K.S. Larsson and H. Boström, *Biol. Neonat. 12*, 41,

20. A. Lahti, E. Antila and L. Saxén, *Teratology 6*, 37, 1972.

21. K.S. Larsson, *Exptl. Cell Research 21*, 498, 1960.

22. K.S. Larsson, *Acta Morphol. Neerl. Scand. 4*, 349, 1962.

23. K.S. Larsson, *Acta Morphol. Neerl. Scand. 4*, 369, 1962.

24. K.S. Larsson, *Acta Odont. Scand. 20,* Suppl. 31, 1962.

25. K.S. Larsson, H. Boström and S. Carlsöö, *Exptl. Cell Research 16,* 379, 1959.

26. K.S. Larsson and E. Cekanova (To be published).

27. C. Lazzaro, *Monit. Zool. Ital. 51,* 249, 1940.

28. A. Levine, S.J. Yaffe and N. Back, *Proc. Soc. Exp. Biol. 129,* 86, 1968.

29. S.Y. Long, K.S. Larsson and S. Lohmander, *Teratology 5,* 261, 1972.

30. L. Marsk, K. Ranning and K.S. Larsson (To be published).

31. L. Marsk, M. Theorell and K.S. Larsson, *Nature 234,* 358, 1971.

32. K.M. Massey, *J. Oral Ther. Pharmacol. 2,* 380, 1966.

33. R. Nanda, *Teratology 3,* 237, 1970.

34. C.E. Nasjleti, J.K. Avery, H.H. Spencer and J.M. Walden, *J. Oral Ther. Pharmacol. 4,* 71, 1967.

35. B.M. Patten, *in* Congenital Anomalies of the Face and Associated Structures, S. Pruzansky (Ed.), Charles C. Thomas, p. 11, 1961.

36. K. Peter, Ergebn. *Anat. Entwickl.- Gesch., 25,* 448, 1924.

37. R.M. Pratt, Jr. (Personal communication).

38. R.M. Pratt, Jr. and C.T.G. King, *Devel. Biol. 27,* 322, 1972.

39. L.M. Ross and B.E. Walker, *Am. J. Anat. 121,* 509, 1967.

40. D.M. Schwartz and A.P. Chaudhry, *J. Dent. Res. 47,* 725, 1968.

41. H. Sicher, *Anat. Anz. 47,* 513, 1915.

42. G.R. Smiley and W.E. Koch, *Anat. Rec. 173,* 405, 1972.

43. A.J. Steffek, A.C. Verrusio and C.A. Watkins, *Teratology 5,* 33, 1972.

44. K. Takano, A.C. Peterson, F.G. Biddle and J.R. Miller, *Teratology 5,* 268, 1972.

45. D.G. Trasler, B.E. Walker and F.C. Fraser, *Science 124,* 439, 1956.

46. A.C. Verrusio, *Teratology 3,* 17, 1970.

47. B.E. Walker, *J. Embryol. Exp. Morph. 9,* 22, 1961.

48. B.E. Walker, *Teratology 4,* 39, 1971.

49. B.E. Walker and F.C. Fraser, *J. Embryol. Exp. Morph. 4,* 176, 1956.

50. B.E. Walker and F.C. Fraser, *J. Embryol. Exp. Morph. 5,* 201, 1957.

51. B.E. Walker and L.M. Ross, *Teratology 5,* 97, 1972.

52. D.H.M. Woolam and J.W. Millen, *in* Ciba Foundation on Congenital Malformations, G.E.W. Wolstenholme and C.M. O'Connor (Eds.), Little, Brown, Boston, p. 158, 1960.

53. L.E. Wragg, M. Klein, G. Steinvorth and R. Warpeha, *Arch. Oral Biol. 15,* 705, 1970.

54. L.E. Wragg, J. Smith and C. Borden, *Anat. Rec. 163,* 288, 1969.

55. E.F. Zimmerman and D. Bowen, *Teratology 5,* 335, 1972.

A SPECIFIC DEVELOPMENTAL DEFECT RELATED TO AN UBIQUITOUS ENZYME: INDUCED MICROMELIA IN THE CHICK EMBRYO TRACEABLE TO DEFECTS IN DEHYDROGENASE AND MOLECULAR ASSEMBLY

Meredith N. Runner

Relatively few major developmental mechanisms or processes in the embryo (Fig. 1) account for normal morphogenesis. These developmental mechanisms are subjected to biochemical regulation at the levels of (a) cellular interactions, (b) synthesis of precursors, (c) transcriptional-translational machinery and (d) post-translational assembly. These regulatory mechanisms of developmental processes are the likely sites of modification by factors inducing congenital malformation.

The following experiments, using 6-Aminonicotinamide (6-AN) as a morphogenetic tool, illustrate the induction of congenital defect resulting from defective post-translational assembly. The observations suggest that alteration of specific chemical reactions, normally occurring in most, if not all, cells can cause specific developmental defects.

Nicotinamide is a derivative of the vitamin, nicotinic acid or niacin (Fig. 2) which is the characteristic subunit for the coenzyme NAD. NAD is a coenzyme for dehydrogenases which can participate in specific anabolic steps and in oxidative phosphorylation, i.e., production of high energy bonds in ATP. The nicotinamide analogue, 6-AN, presumably becomes assembled into a false NAD, resulting in deficiency of certain dehydrogenase reactions which in turn produces teratogenesis. Although 6-AN is believed to act at these very specific biochemical reactions, dehydrogenases are ubiquitous. Additional information is needed to account for the observed embryonic specificity of effects, i.e., micromelia.

The reality of biochemical specificity of action of 6-AN has been demonstrated by protection from severe micromelia with the normal counterpart, nicotinamide (Fig. 3). Protection from micromelia is afforded when nicotinamide is administered prior to or simultaneously with 6-AN. The loss of capability to rescue from or to reverse the effects of 6-AN is detectible within 1 hour after administering 6-AN. It is apparent that, as 6-AN becomes bound, the effectiveness of nicotinamide to rescue from micromelia diminishes. These observations on protection, competition and reversibility *in vivo*

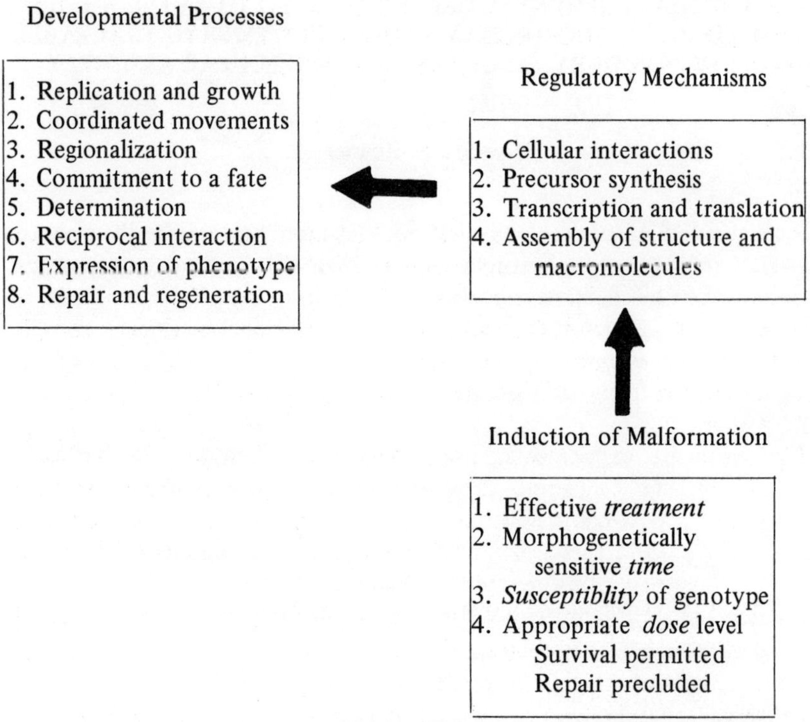

Developmental Processes

1. Replication and growth
2. Coordinated movements
3. Regionalization
4. Commitment to a fate
5. Determination
6. Reciprocal interaction
7. Expression of phenotype
8. Repair and regeneration

Regulatory Mechanisms

1. Cellular interactions
2. Precursor synthesis
3. Transcription and translation
4. Assembly of structure and
     macromolecules

Induction of Malformation

1. Effective *treatment*
2. Morphogenetically
     sensitive *time*
3. *Susceptiblity* of genotype
4. Appropriate *dose* level
     Survival permitted
     Repair precluded

Fig. 1. Perspectives in teratogenesis. Major developmental processes which account for embryogenesis and morphogenesis come under regulatory controls which are probable sites of action of teratogens. A teratogenic agent in order to be effective must meet all 4 of the prerequisites: treatment, time, susceptibility and dose (TTSD).

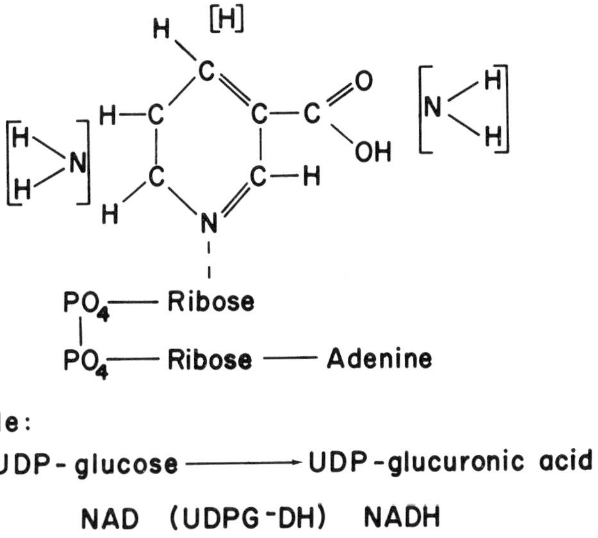

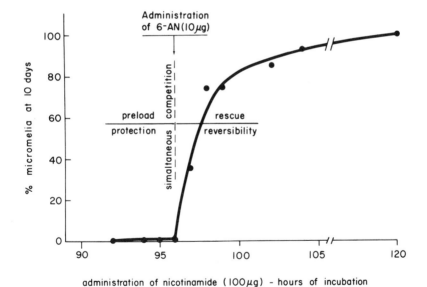

Fig. 2. Formula for nicotinic acid and derivatives; nicotinamide (niacin), 6-aminonicotinamide (6-AN) and nicotinamide adenine dinucleotide (DPN or NAD).

Fig. 3. Protection, competition, reversibility experiments. Nicotinamide (100 μg.) was administered at various times before, after and concomitant with 6-aminonicotinamide (10 μg). Each point represents the mean of 30 to 40 embryos. Adapted from Overman *et al.,* 1972.

demonstrate the biochemical specificity of 6-AN to participate as an analogue of nicotinamide.

A pedigree of events associated with chondrodystrophy or micromelia begins with synthesis of chondroitin sulfate. Glucose, amino acids and sulfate are required as precursors (Fig. 4). Glucose is converted to unusual hexose sugars, namely galactosamine and glucuronic acid, which occur in characteristic proportions in chondroitin sulfate. Amino acids are synthesized into a core protein to which the hexose side chains, made up from galactosamine and glucuronic acid, are attached. Cellular organelles synthesize core protein on ribosomes attached to the rough endoplasmic reticulum (Fig. 5). While the nascent polypeptide chains remain attached to the ribosomes and the membranes of the RER, some of the hexose sugars are attached. Completion of attachment of sugars to the protein occurs after the endoplasmic reticulum has become smooth. The resulting mucopolysaccharide is transported to the Golgi apparatus where sulfation of galactosamine occurs. The completely assembled molecules are then transported outside the cell by Golgi vesicles. The product, chondroitin sulfate is a main component of cartilaginous matrix.

Experiments using labeled amino acids and glucosamine suggest that under the influence of 6-AN the chick limb bud shows a reduced amount of sulfate incorporation[1] at a time when amino acids and glucosamine are used in normal quantities. It appears that in the presence of 6-AN, protein core and hexose side chains are assembled but the molecule remains incompletely sulfated.

Both the morphological observations[2] and the inhibition of incorporation of ^{35}S-sulfate[3] indicate subnormal quantity of the special product, chondroitin sulfate. Perhaps there is a failure to deliver mucopolysaccharide to the Golgi apparatus. Perhaps there is enzyme inhibition which precludes sulfation. In any event, the morphological and biochemical effects are detectible 24 hours after administering 6-AN to 96-hour embryos. Products accumulate in the endoplasmic reticulum of chondrogenic cells. The Golgi do not become enlarged as they normally should. Since assembly of the chondroitin sulfate molecule is incomplete and export is inhibited by 6-AN, the typical intercellular matrix in the chondrogenic area fails to appear. (Biochemical repair can be seen after two or three days[2] but by this time the cartilage model is misshapen and ossification employs an abnormal cartilaginous model.) The result is micromelia.

The experiments using 6-AN suggest a highly localized effect of a drug specifically on chondrocytes within limb buds of the embryo. One hypothesis to explain the localized specificity postulates existence of compartmental or regional sensitivity to 6-AN on the part of chondrogenic cells of the limb. For example, specific reactions which produce the energy bonds for synthesis of

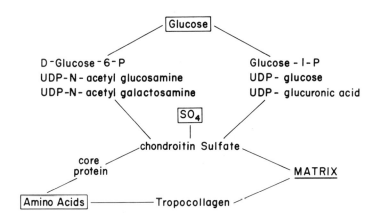

Fig. 4. Diagram of assembly of chondroitin sulfate showing precursor components glucose (galactosamine and glucuronic acid), amino acids and sulfate.

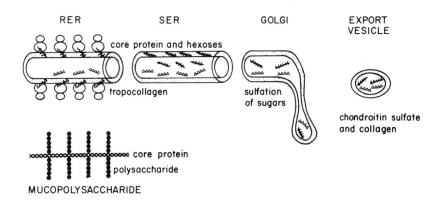

Fig. 5. Scheme showing sites of assembly and export of chondroitin sulfate. Based on Seegmiller *et al.*, 1972.

mucopolysaccharides in the limb may be selectively inhibited by abnormal cofactor. Perhaps dehydrogenase enzymes in these sensitive regions have receptor sites with greater-than-usual affinity for abnormal cofactor. This hypothesis suggests a selective or qualitative effect of 6-AN. Another hypothesis postulates a differential consequence of generalized inhibition of dehydrogenase by 6-AN. Although all dehydrogenase reactions may be impaired, those reactions requiring the presence of large quantities of NAD for mass production of macromolecules, viz. chondroitin sulfate, may be the first to exhibit effects of an increased quantity of abnormal NAD. Constitutive products essential for subsistence of cells may be produced without inter-ruption because their dehydrogenases exist with a margin of safety or because they require lower concentrations of normal NAD cofactor. Inter-ruption of synthesis and export of so-called luxury molecules would have less margin of safety and inhibition would be highly visible. The 4-day chick limb shows that inhibition of intercellular matrix is the predominant effect of 6-AN. The data do not permit a clear distinction between the qualitative and quantitative hypotheses to account for localized specificity.

The pursuit of precise mechanisms by which teratogens produce congenital abnormalities has been rewarding but explanations remain incomplete. The new knowledge about transitory achondrogenesis in the embryonic limb, is that 6-AN causes enlargement of the endoplasmic reticulum, under develop-ment of the Golgi and incomplete assembly of chondroitin sulfate. It has been shown that the site of inhibition and the cause of atypical morphogenesis is at the assembly of a specialized produce, chondroitin sulfate, normally in large quantities. It is understandable that, in the absence of appropriate quantities of cartilaginous matrix, atypical bone is formed and that the outcome is micromelia. Additional experiments are needed to determine which specific reactions, involving NAD as dehydrogenase coenzyme, are accountable for incomplete assembly of chondroitin sulfate molecules. Additional experiments are needed to explain the localized response to 6-AN.

6-AN is an example of a post-translational teratogen which has its effect on the assembly of precursors. A deficiency of completed chondroitin sulfate molecules, normally produced in large quantity in a localized part of the embryonic limb bud, is created. Such studies on micromelia induced by 6-AN have contributed toward a deeper understanding of morphogenesis and teratogenesis.

The experiments indicate (a) the biochemical specificity of a teratogen, like 6-AN, because the consequences stem from a false coenzyme, 6-AN-NAD, and (b) the highly specific effect on molecular assembly within the embryonic limb irrespective of the ubiquity of a family of enzymes (dehydrogenases) which are modifiable by the teratogen.

It will be important to learn whether the teratogenic agent lowered the effectiveness of all dehydrogenase reactions or whether certain enzymatic steps, critical in chondrogenesis, are particularly sensitive to the false cofactor. The possibility exists that an environmental teratogen can lower reaction rates of a family of enzymes and yet produce specific malformations. Environmental factors having generalized metabolic effects, therefore, can serve as teratogenic agents (see Fig. 1) when an effective dose impinges upon a genetically susceptible embryo at a sensitive time in development.

REFERENCES

1. D.O. Overman, R.E. Seegmiller and M.N. Runner, *Dev. Biol. 28*, 573, 1972.

2. R.E. Seegmiller, D.O. Overman and M.N. Runner, *Dev. Biol. 28*, 555, 1972.

3. R.E. Seegmiller and M.N. Runner, *J. Emb. Exp. Morph.* (in press).

ACKNOWLEDGEMENTS

This work was supported by grants from the National Institutes of Health, National Institute of Child Health and Human Development (HD 02282) and from the National Science Foundation (GB 14662). Special thanks are extended to Mrs. Karen Howard and Miss Susan McAferty for technical assistance.

DISCUSSION

DR. BECKER: Dr. Larsson, how does a compound which is given on day 10 and which falls below detectable levels in the embryo on day 11 produce cleft palate by day 14½ or day 15? Also, some compounds, diazepam and diphenylhydantoin are good examples, produce two peaks of cleft palate. One of these is on day 12 while the other occurs on days 14–15, close to the actual events of palate closure. Could you suggest the possible mechanisms for these two events?

DR. LARSSON: I think this is a difficult question to answer. I have never designed an experiment or tried it in that way. It could be possible, as suggested by Zimmerman for glucocorticoids, that these compounds are interfering with the production of DNA or RNA within the palatine shelves. Thus, some of the enzymes essential for later development could be affected long before the event of palate closure.

DR. SKALKO: The halogenated deoxyuridines, which are incorporated into DNA, are incapable of producing cleft palate beyond day 11. Dr. Becker's point is an important one, namely, to recognize the limits of resolution of our experimental methods. We are incapable of detecting these, and related teratogens, at a certain point in time after administration even though the morphogenetic processes that these compounds affect occur much later. There are two possible explanations: either we've exceeded the limits of resolution so that the compounds are still there but we don't see them or, in classical terms, we have altered the "prospective fate" of these cells irreversibly and the compound does not have to be there anymore. It is important to recognize that we are dealing with developing systems and I think that this is where the difference between toxicity and teratogenicity is important.

DR. PORTER: You made an interesting observation about the possibility that there may be two stem lines present in the embryo and they might have differential effects on your particular study. Where did you get the idea that there might be two different cell lines and in what way are they different?

DR. SKALKO: The concept of sensitive and tolerant cells comes from the tissue culture literature. In general, two types of cells have been described with respect to their response to bromodeoxyuridine, those which are sensitive and those which are resistant. The resistant cell lines have a mutation at the locus controlling thymidine kinase. They don't incorporate BUdR into DNA and are not sensitive to its action. Other investigators have described cells which incorporate BUdR, but there are no discernable biological effects. The definition of tolerant cells, then, is an operational one derived from the observation that not all cells which incorporate BUdR express an observable biological effect. All of the autoradiographic data which I reviewed revealed no preferential localization of any compound. This makes it intellectually unsatisfying when you're dealing with very specific tissue responses unless you postulate that there are two populations which cannot be discriminated from each other: one which is sensitive and one which is tolerant.

DR. NANCE: I'd like to ask Dr. Runner if any phenocopies of the 6-aminonicotinamide chick have been studied with respect to nicotinamide metabolism. It seems to me that this has been an exciting area to try and see whether known genetic mutants are analogs of teratogenic models.

DR. RUNNER: The answer is an unsatisfactory yes. Ursula Abbott and her group at Davis, California have a number of mutants of limb development and these mutants have been and are being studied in relation to these various analogs. The answer you would really like has not been done but I think it is on the way.

DR. PORTER: Are there any members of the panel or of the audience who are aware of any studies of the genetic determination of dilantin excretion in animals? There is, as you know, some evidence that dilantin excretion may be genetically determined in man.

DR. BECKER: As well as I recall, the major metabolite of diphenylhydantoin is hydroxyphenylhydantoin in man, dog, rabbit, rat and mouse, but the kinetics are not uniform. In the rat and dog they are extremely rapid and the mouse is extremely slow; in man they are somewhere in between. Recently, another metabolite which may be extremely important to man has been described, the dihydro derivative. This derivative is found in man to quite an appreciable extent, somewhat less so in the dog and I am not sure about the mouse. In any event, this metabolite appears to play a greater role in man than in other animals. As far as excretion is concerned, the half-life of diphenylhydantoin in man is approximately 12 hours, in the order of 6 to 8 hours in the rat and about 14 to 16 hours in the mouse.

OVERVIEW

Abraham M. Lilienfeld

To provide an overview of this productive and stimulating meeting in which a variety of pertinent and relevant problems have been discussed, I decided to approach the task by taking an overview of the major objective of this symposium — New Directions to be Taken in Birth Defects. I would like to orient my comments primarily to those broad areas covered by the speakers, particularly with regard to some problems within these areas, rather than summarize with a few specific remarks and general comments, the papers presented or areas covered. At the same time, I will try to indicate some of the new directions that have been proposed in the papers presented and the discussions that followed.

I think that the areas covered by this symposium can be considered as follows:

1. Population studies; papers by Neel, Rush and Newcombe fall into this category.
2. Effects of maternal factors.
3. Mechanisms of actions of teratogens.
4. Policy or program considerations, including problems of monitoring or surveillance, experimental testing of potential teratogens, problems in prevention such as rubella vaccination and cost benefit analysis.

In selecting subjects for consideration within these areas, I will allow my biases to play a role and I will attempt to be selective in order to protect you from exposure to another detailed paper.

In the discussion of population studies, many differences of opinion were presented. If one believes that there is a general overall constancy in the frequency of malformations in different countries or in different regions of a country where considerable variation in environmental conditions exist, such as diet, occupational exposures, climatic conditions, etc., then one might think, as Neel does, that malformations are caused principally by "the intrinsic properties of multigenic Mendelian inheritance."

However, before one can make this inference, it is rather important to assess the frequency of the population data with which one is dealing. I attempted to do this several years ago and found that the published literature was most difficult to comprehend.[1] There are differences in the types of conditions that are included in any one series as compared to another. At today's symposium, this became rather striking when the list of conditions shown by Newcombe is contrasted with those usually reported by Neel. However, even if similar conditions are included in the categories, there remain the problems of diagnosis where a great deal of variability clearly persists. Different conditions are defined differently by different investigators although they are similarly named.

It is of interest that even though Neel emphasized similarities in frequency, the actual data presented at the symposium clearly showed several differences. For example, the data on anencephaly and spina bifida indicated that they were much higher in Wales than in Israel — almost 4-fold.

The importance of determining more definitively whether there really are differences in the frequency of malformations in different populations was illustrated by the important inferences in Renwick's presentation of the possible influence of blighted potatoes on anencephaly. Although he did not want to directly attribute causation to this relationship, it's a question of semantics since the inference was that potato abstention can only be based upon a causal relationship. I personally am not as convinced as he is regarding the potential of prevention, but it is an exciting hypothesis requiring further testing as Dr. Renwick proposes.

The presentations concerned with this area clearly suggest some new directions. There is an urgent need for the standardization of definitions of the different forms of malformations as well as the development of diagnostic criteria. In addition, I think that it would be highly desirable to develop on an international basis and on a regional basis within the United States, 12 to 20 collaborating centers where examinations of infants can be carried out in a standardized and rigorously controlled manner so that population frequencies can be provided for comparisons. This suggestion also pertains to the entire issue of monitoring.

In comparing population groups, we must not fail to remember that the malformations which we detect actually represent the "top of the iceberg;" there is much that lies below in the form of early and late fetal death. Thus, even if we note similarities in frequency, there may well be differences that lie lurking beneath the observed water level. It may, therefore, be essential to obtain standardized estimates of this remaining spectrum which could be quite important in elucidating the presence of environmental teratogens.

Another population subgroup that has received some consideration is twins. All of us have experienced difficulties with twin studies. To date, they have not really provided the clear-cut answers that were promised decades ago.

However, one new direction which does have promise and should be actively pursued is the one outlined by Nance, who suggests studying the offspring of monozygotic twins. This is a most intriguing idea, although I must admit that operationally it could be quite difficult. Nevertheless, I think the potential results appear sufficiently promising to warrant the effort.

Another type of population study was suggested by the presentation of Janerich whose analysis pointed toward studies of the young mother, i.e., those under 20 years of age giving birth to anencephalic children. I think that his very neat cohort analysis strongly suggests the need for studying the characteristics of young mothers of anencephalics and a control group − in addition to potato consumption. Perhaps such studies should be done for all types of birth defects.

One of the most interesting recent findings has been that of the prenatally administered stilbesterol induced vaginal or cervical cancer reviewed by Greenwald. This certainly has tremendous implications since it indicates that the transplacental transmission of a chemical can produce an effect after a lengthy latent or incubation period. To this should be added the possibility that influenza infection during pregnancy may increase the risk of leukemia in the offspring as recently reported in the British Medical Journal.[2] If events during pregnancy have this long range effect, it becomes essential to determine what components of diet as well as of infections, drugs and other environmental agents might have on the developing human organism in general. Although we have for many years emphasized such maternal effects with respect to malformations and brain damage, at this point obviously other diseases should be included. This entire area requires the addition of a new dimension to our investigative effort.

Perhaps these effects can be determined by measuring morphologic variants as suggested by Hook. These variants may be part of the submerged part of the iceberg, thereby indicating another research direction. If this is so, it is quite possible that the long term follow-up studies one ordinarily depends upon to elucidate such effects may not be necessary.

At the policy-making level, one of the major issues discussed at the symposium was the relationship of the results of animal testing for teratogens to humans. A more systematic study of the comparative effects of teratogens in animals with that in humans is certainly in order. From what I have been able to gather − a great deal of work needs to be done in systematic comparisons.

The problems associated with this area and the potential for new directions were quite amply covered and are still fresh in our minds; anything I might add would be superfluous. But, the discussion did emphasize the need for human studies and Newcombe's suggestion for following a consecutive series of individuals receiving the first 100,000 prescriptions for a new drug does point

287

in a new direction. I hope his suggestion does not go unexplored.

Experimental work on mechanisms of action of agents are important from the viewpoint of human studies and not merely from a puristic viewpoint since once a mechanism can be found in an animal, it can be looked for in humans and thereby provide an improved method of screening drugs as emphasized by Layton. There is no need to indicate the implications of his exposition of differences in pharmacokinetics, metabolism of placenta and embryo, etc. These also point to new directions; it isn't clear, however, how operational this viewpoint is in the absence of adequate data on metabolism.

I think it's obvious from the presentations and discussions that there are several new directions for investigative work, in animal experiments and human population areas. Many of the studies I have mentioned are not easy to execute – they are more difficult than those we have been doing; but, as one poet said, "Ah, but a man's reach should exceed his grasp, or what's a Heaven for?"

REFERENCES

1. A.M. Lilienfeld, *in* Proceedings of the Third International Conference on Congenital Malformations, F.C. Fraser, V.A. McKusick and R. Robinson (Eds.), Excerpta Medica, International Congress Series No. 204, New York, p. 251, 1970.

2. J. Fedrick and E.D. Alberman, *Brit. Med. J. 2,* 485, 1972.

AUTHOR'S NOTE

This symposium was both interesting and exciting. I would like to take this opportunity to personally thank Dr. Janerich, our symposium organizer; his committee; the Birth Defects Institute at the New York State Department of Health, particularly Dr. Porter; those who presented papers; and the audience for participating in two enjoyable and stimulating days.

SUBJECT INDEX

A

Abortion, 131, 220, 221
  spontaneous, 134
  therapeutic, 133, 134
Acetazolamide, 212, 213, 214
Achondroplastic dwarf, 12, 35
Acid-soluble fractions, 242
Actinomycin, 239
Active transport, 206
Acute leukemias, 197
Acute toxicity, 196
Adenocarcinoma, 159, 160
Adrenal cancers, 152
Adrenal tumors, 156
Aflatoxins, 51
Alcohol (consumption), 174, 176, 179,
  183
American Academy of Pediatrics, 136
American Association of Health Data
  Systems, 127
Amethopterin, 197
6-Aminonicotinamide, 19, 250, 264, 267,
  275, 284
Aminopterin, 197, 227
Amniotic cavity, 207
Amniotic fluid, 264
Amniotic puncture, 267
Anencephaly, 6, 9, 21, 73, 113, 185, 189,
  190, 192, 286, *see also* Epidemics
  and spina bifida, 186
Aqueductal stenosis, 219
Arthralgia, 133
Ascites, 221
Aspirin, 210, 212, 230, 231
Atresia ani, 9
Autoradiography, 239, 246, 258
6-Azauridine, 239

B

Behavioral studies, 199
β-Hemolytic streptococcus, 10

Benzoic acid, 210, 238
Betamethasone, 260
Biotransformation, 207, 208, 209, 212,
  214, 227, 230
  of drugs, 207
  of steroid hormones, 207
Birth order, 75, 99, *see also* Parity
Birthweight, 161–183
Bladder, 155
  cancers of, 152
  tumors of, 156
Blood levels, 230
Blue Tongue virus, 220
Breast tumors, 156
Bromodeoxyuridine, 283
British Columbia Registry of Handicapped
  Children and Adults, 96
BUdR, 239, 242, 246

C

Caffeine, 212
Cartilaginous matrix, 278
Cataracts, 131, 132
Carbonic anhydrase, 214
  inhibitors, 214
Cell
  death, 208
  division, 208
  migration, 208
  products, 250
  shapes, 208
  types, 246
Center for Disease Control, 123, 133
Central nervous system, 199, 219, 220,
  224
  defect, 4
Cephalometric, 26
Cerebellar hypoplasia, 224
Cervical adenocarcinoma, 150
Cervix, 159
Chaconines, 186
Chick embryo, 214

289